# ATLAS OF PALPATORY ANATOMY OF THE LOWER EXTREMITIES

# ATLAS OF PALPATORY ANATOMY OF THE LOWER EXTREMITIES

## A MANUAL INSPECTION OF THE SURFACE

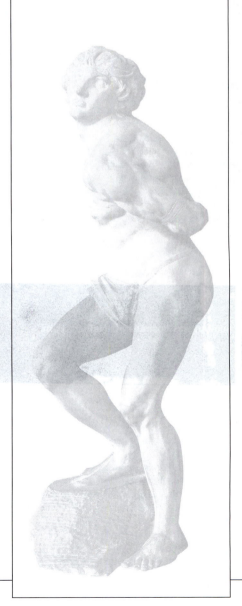

## SERGE TIXA

Teacher in Anatomy and in Palpatory Anatomy
Swiss School of Osteopathy of Lausanne
Lausanne, Switzerland

Translated by
## NORMAND MILLER, M.D., FRCSC

Director, Vascular Laboratory
Mercy Medical Center
Baltimore, Maryland

Illustrations by
Holly R. Fischer, MFA

Ann Arbor, Michigan

McGraw-Hill, Inc.
Health Professions Division

New York   St. Louis   San Francisco   Auckland   Bogotá
Caracas   Lisbon   London   Madrid   Mexico City   Milan   Montreal
New Delhi   San Juan   Singapore   Sydney   Tokyo   Toronto

**McGraw-Hill**

*A Division of The* **McGraw·Hill** *Companies*

ATLAS OF PALPATORY ANATOMY
OF THE LOWER EXTREMITIES

1234567890 DOCDOC 99


ISBN 0-07-065357-7


This book was set in Times Roman by York Graphic Services.
The editors were John Dolan and Muza Navrozov.
The production supervisor was Helene G. Landers.
The text and cover were designed by Marsha Cohen / Parallelogram Graphics.
The index was prepared by Edwin Durban.
R. R. Donnelley and Sons Company was printer and binder.

This book is printed on acid-free paper.




Originally published as *Atlas d'anatomie palpatoire du membre inférieur.
Investigation manuelle de surface,* © Masson, Paris 1997


Michaelangelo illustration © Nathan, Paris.




Library of Congress Cataloging-in-Publication Data
Tixa, Serge
        [Atlas d'anatomie palpatoire du membre inferieur. English]
        Atlas of palpatory anatomy of the lower extremities : a manual
inspection of the surface / Serge Tixa ; translated from the French
by Normand Miller ; illustrations by Holly R. Fischer.
            p. cm.
        Includes index.
        ISBN 0-07-065357-7
        1. Leg—Anatomy—Atlases. 2. Hip joint—Anatomy—Atlases. 3. Anatomy, Surgical and topographical—Atlases. I. Title
    QM549 .T5913 1999
    611'.98'0222—dc21

# CONTENTS

**Preface to the English Edition**   ix

**Introduction**   xi

## PART I. THE HIP

Illustrated Study oateral)   2
Illustrated Study of the Hip (Posterior)   3
Topographic Presentation of the Hip   4

### Chapter 1. Osteology   5

The Iliofemoral Region   5
The Iliac Bone   6
The Femur   10

### Chapter 2. Myology   13

The Lateral Inguinofemoral Region   13
The Medial Inguinofemoral Region
or Femoral Triangle   15
The Gluteal Region   18
  Superficial Plane   19
  Middle Plane   21
  Deep Plane   23

### Chapter 3. Nerves and Vessels   28

The Medial Inguinofemoral Region or
Scarpa's Triangle   28
The Gluteal Region   30
  The Greater Sciatic Nerve   30

## PART II. THE THIGH

Illustrated Study of the Thigh (Anterior)   34
Illustrated Study of the Thigh (Posterior)   34
Illustrated Study of the Thigh (Lateral)   35
Illustrated Study of the Thigh (Medial)   35

Topographic Presentation
of the Thigh (Femur)   36

### Chapter 4. Myology   37

The Anterofemoral Region: The Anterior
Muscular Group   37
  The Sartorius Muscle   38
  The Quadriceps Extensor Muscle   40
  Tensor Muscle of the Fascia Lata   43
The Posterofemoral Region   45

The Medial Muscular Group   46
  The Adductor Muscles   47
  The Gracilis Muscle   49
The Posterior Muscular Group   51
  The Medial Hamstring Muscles   52
  The Lateral Hamstring Muscle   55

## PART III. THE KNEE

Illustrated Study of the Knee (Anterior)   58
Illustrated Study of the Knee (Posterior)   58
Illustrated Study of the Knee (Lateral)   59
Illustrated Study of the Knee (Medial)   59

Topographic Presentation of the Knee   60

### Chapter 5. Osteology   61

The Anterior Compartment   61
The Medial Compartment   66
The External Compartment   70

### Chapter 6. Arthrology: The Articulations   75

The Ligaments   75

### Chapter 7. Myology   81

The Anterolateral Region   81
  The Thigh   82
  The Leg   83
The Anteromedial Region   85
The Posterior Region   90

### Chapter 8. Nerves and Vessels   93

The Popliteal Fossa   93
  The Tibial Nerve   94
  The Peroneal Nerve   96
  The Sural Nerve   97
  The Popliteal Artery   98

## PART IV. THE LEG

Illustrated Study of the Lower Leg (Anterior)   100
Illustrated Study of the Lower Leg (Posterior)   100
Illustrated Study of the Lower Leg (Lateral)   101
Illustrated Study of the Lower Leg (Medial)   101

Topographic Presentation of the Leg   102

### Chapter 9. Osteology   103

Leg   103

**Chapter 10. Myology   105**

The Anterior Muscular Group   105
  The Anterior Tibialis Muscle   106
  The Extrinsic Extensor Muscles of the Toes
  and the Peroneus Tertius Muscle   108
The Lateral Muscular Group   111
  The Peroneus Longus Muscle   112
  The Peroneus Brevis Muscle   114
  The Posterior Muscular Group   116
  The Superficial Plane   117
    The Triceps Surae Muscle and the Plantaris Muscle   117
  Deep Plane   122
    The Posterior Tibialis Muscle   122
    The Flexor Digitorum Longus Muscle   124
    The Flexor Hallucis Longus Muscle   126

**PART V. THE ANKLE AND FOOT**

Illustrated Study of the Ankle/Foot (Anterior)   130
Illustrated Study of the Ankle/Foot (Dorsum)   130
Illustrated Study of the Ankle/Foot (Lateral)   131
Illustrated Study of the Ankle/Foot (Medial)   131

Topographic Presentation of the Foot   132

**Chapter 11. Osteology   133**

The Lateral Border   133
  The Fifth Metatarsal Bone   134
  The Cuboid Bone   136
  The Calcaneus   137
  The Talus   140
  The Lateral Malleolus   141
The Medial Border   142
  The First Metatarsal Bone   143
  The Medial Cuneiform Bone   146
  The Navicular Bone   147

The Talus   148
The Calcaneus   150
The Medial Malleolus   151
The Anterior Surface of the Ankle and the Dorsal Surface
of the Foot   152
The Posterior Surface of the Ankle and of the Foot   156
The Plantar Surface   159

**Chapter 12. Arthrology   164**

The Articulations   164
  The Articular Interspaces and the Ligaments   164
  The Interphalangeal Joints   165
  The Metatarsophalangeal Joints   166
  The Articulation of Lisfranc
  or the Tarsometatarsal Joints   167
  The Articulation of Chopart or the Medial Tarsal Joint   169
  The Posterior Calcaneotalar or Subtalar Joint
  and the Anterior Calcaneotalar Joint   170
  The Tibiotarsal Joint   171
  The Ligaments of the Tibiotarsal Joint   173
  The Posteroinferior Tibiofibular Ligament   175
  The Annular Ligaments of the Tarsum and the Dorsal
  Aponeurosis of the Foot   175

**Chapter 13. Myology   177**

The Musculotendinous Structures of the Ankle and the Foot   177
The Intrinsic Muscles of the Foot   184

**Chapter 14. Nerves and Vessels   191**

**Bibliography   195**

**Index   197**

**Notes   207**

# PREFACE TO THE ENGLISH EDITION

Professor Tixa's book *Atlas of Palpatory Anatomy of the Lower Extremities* is an important tool for students and beginning clinicians in understanding normal anatomy. While the book is not meant to replace the broader illustrated textbooks of anatomy, it does serve as a unique supplement in presenting quality photographs along with other visual clues for determining the major muscles, nerves, ligaments, and tendons of the lower extremities.

Students in physical therapy, occupational therapy, podiatry, and medicine as well as other students learning anatomy will find this Atlas a valuable resource for use in training and in their professional career. In addition, beginning clinicians doing physical assessments will find the book as a good review.

In this English edition, line art has been added to the opening of each section. Most students initially learn anatomy through line art, and the student thus will not have to turn to another source for this type of review. It is the quality and detail of the photographs, though, that students should get the most benefit from.

The publisher wishes to thank Dr. Normand Miller for his translation of the original French text into English; Holly Fischer, MFA, for her superb illustrations; and Richard Wilcox, for his initial development work.

In addition, we gratefully acknowledge the following for their critical reviews and suggestions on the manuscript: Paul A. Anderson, Ph.D., (Department of Physical Therapy, School of Medicine, University of Maryland, Baltimore, Maryland) and David Garrison, Ph.D. (Department of Physical Therapy, University of Oklahoma Health Sciences Center, Oklahoma City, Oklahoma).

Professor Tixa is completing an *Atlas of the Upper Extremities,* and we hope to bring that out as a second volume in the very near future.

McGraw-Hill
January, 1999

# INTRODUCTION

This book represents a method of ("palpatory") surface anatomy (or "anatomy of palpation"); it is based on the manual inspection of surface forms (MISF), a visual and didactic method of investigating the anatomic structures (bones, ligaments, tendons, muscles, nerves, and vessels). Each structure is illustrated by a photograph, which is accompanied by text describing the technique of approach to the illustrated structure.

## For Whom Is It Intended?

For those who require a method of applied anatomy in the practice of their profession.

## How Is the Book Organized?

This book includes 385 photographs of the lower extremities; it is divided into five parts, focusing on the hip, thigh, knee, calf, ankle, and foot. As appropriate to the given topographic area, each part is further subdivided into the following sections: Osteology, Myology (or musculotendinous structures), Arthrology (joints and ligaments), and Nerves and Vessels.

There are two types of photographs.

- Photographs of presentation:
  –General presentation, introducing a part (Hip—Thigh—Calf—Ankle—Foot).
  –Topographic presentation, showing a comprehensive view of a region with structures accessible to palpation (e.g., the lateral inguinofemoral region or the lateral border of the foot).
  –Structural presentation, illustrating, when possible, the anatomic structure and its relationships with the adjacent structures. These are mainly presentations of muscles or muscular groups (e.g., the quadriceps extensor muscle).

- MISF photographs:
  –The essential part of this work, visualizing the investigated structure and describing the technique of approach.

## How to Use It?

There are two possible methods:

- To study a region (e.g., the knee) or part of a region (e.g., the lateral border of the foot) thoroughly, refer to the part or chapter of interest in the Table of Contents.
- To study a specific structure from all possible angles, refer to the Index, which lists all photographs related to the subject (e.g., the sartorius muscle is dealt with in Part II, "The Thigh," as well as Parts I and III, "The Hip" and "The Knee").

*Comment:*

- The delimitation of the regions studied in each part should not be interpreted too strictly, since some muscles, for example, will extend beyond the areas of emphasis. This is justified by the fact that each muscle is studied not only in a transverse approach, in relation to the adjacent structures, but also longitudinally in terms of its origin, body, and site of insertion (e.g., the iliopsoas muscle, which extends far beyond the medial inguinofemoral region, found also in the abdominal region).
- In the text, the hand or grip of the examiner is often labeled "proximal" or "distal," depending on whether it is moving closer to or further away from the origin of the leg being examined.

# ATLAS OF PALPATORY ANATOMY OF THE LOWER EXTREMITIES

# THE HIP

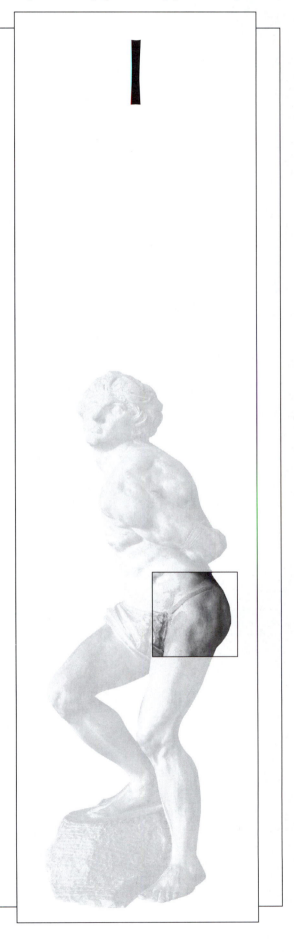

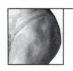
# ILLUSTRATED STUDY OF THE HIP (LATERAL)

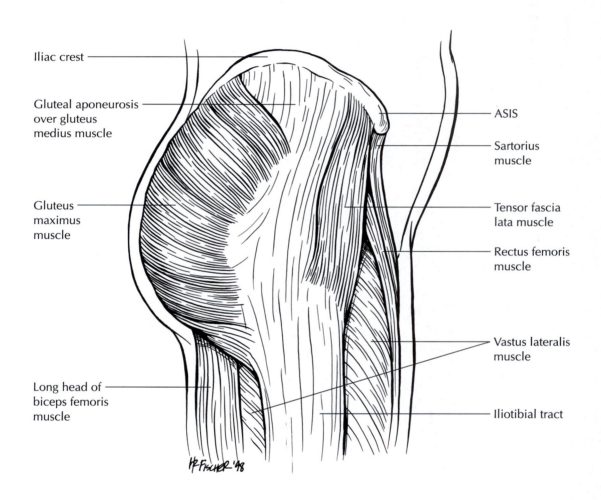

Iliac crest

Gluteal aponeurosis over gluteus medius muscle

Gluteus maximus muscle

Long head of biceps femoris muscle

ASIS

Sartorius muscle

Tensor fascia lata muscle

Rectus femoris muscle

Vastus lateralis muscle

Iliotibial tract

# ILLUSTRATED STUDY OF THE HIP (POSTERIOR)

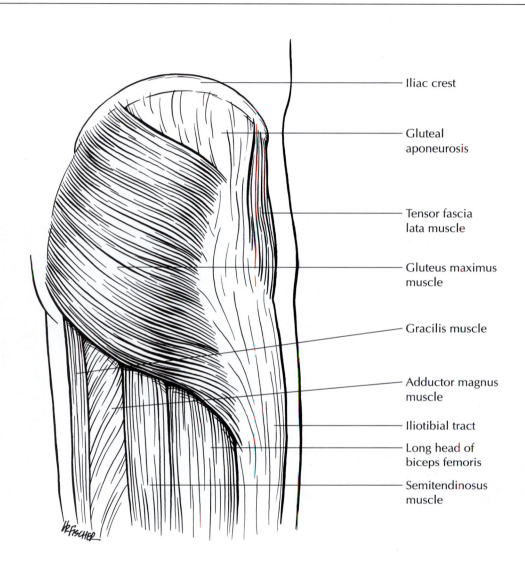

Iliac crest

Gluteal aponeurosis

Tensor fascia lata muscle

Gluteus maximus muscle

Gracilis muscle

Adductor magnus muscle

Iliotibial tract

Long head of biceps femoris

Semitendinosus muscle

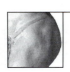 

## TOPOGRAPHIC PRESENTATION OF THE HIP

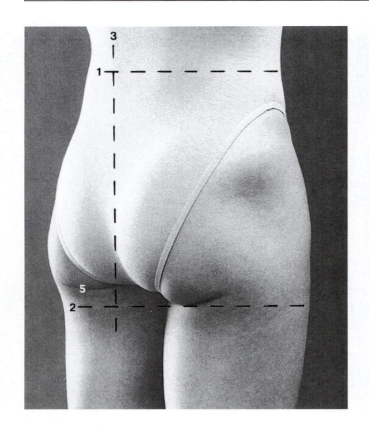

**FIGURE 1-1**
**POSTEROLATERAL VIEW**

1. Superior border
2. Inferior border
3. Posteromedial border

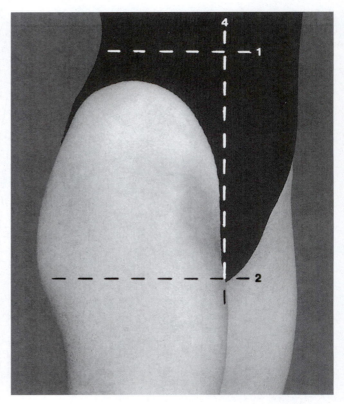

**FIGURE 1-2**
**ANTEROLATERAL VIEW**

4. Anteromedial border
5. Gluteal fold

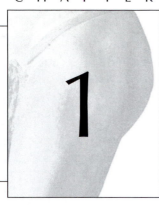

# 1

# OSTEOLOGY

## THE ILIOFEMORAL REGION

The bony structures accessible by palpation are as follows below.

### The Iliac Bone:

- the iliac crest (Fig. 1-4)
- the anterosuperior iliac spine (Fig. 1-5)
- the tubercle of the iliac crest (Fig. 1-6)
- the pubic tubercle (Fig. 1-7)
- the posterosuperior iliac spine (Fig. 1-8)
- the small "coxal notch" (Fig. 1-9)
- the posteroinferior iliac spine (Fig. 1-9)

- the ischial spine (Fig. 1-10)
- the lesser sciatic notch (Fig. 1-10)
- the greater sciatic notch (Fig. 1-11)
- the ischial tuberosity (Fig. 1-12)
- the inferior border of the iliac bone (Fig. 1-13)

### The Femur:

- the femoral head (Figs. 1-14, 1-15, and 1-16)
- the greater trochanter (Figs. 1-17 and 1-18)
- the lesser trochanter (Figs. 1-19 and 1-20)

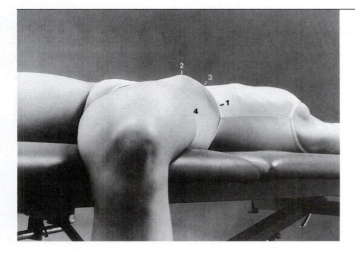

**FIGURE 1-3**

**LOW-ANGLE VIEW OF THE HIP REGION**

*(THE PATIENT IS SUPINE; THE KNEE IS IN THE FOREGROUND)*

*ILIAC BONE*

1. Iliac crest
2. Anterosuperior iliac spine
3. Tubercle of the iliac crest

*FEMUR*

4. Greater trochanter

# THE ILIAC BONE

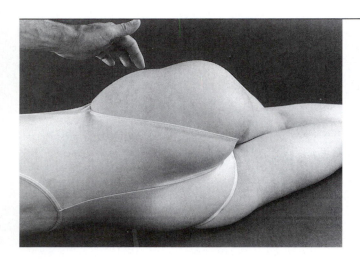

### FIGURE 1-4
#### THE ILIAC CREST

It is possible to perceive changes in the curvature of this structure as well as its variations in thickness. To do so, follow it from front to back and from back to front using bidigital palpation or grabbing it between your thumb and index finger.

The crest itself as well as its lateral and medial "borders" should be followed.

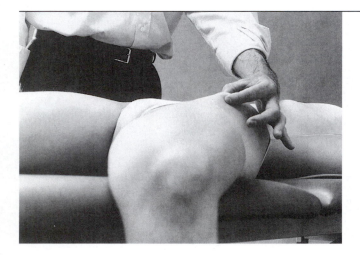

### FIGURE 1-5
#### THE ANTEROSUPERIOR ILIAC SPINE

This is easy to access. Begin by finding the precise location of the most anterior part of the iliac crest. Grab this structure between your thumb and index finger to delineate it clearly.

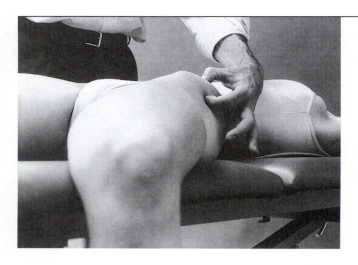

### FIGURE 1-6
#### THE TUBERCLE OF THE ILIAC CREST

Located on top of the anterior curvature, this structure projects toward the external iliac fossa. Follow the iliac crest from front to back between your thumb and index finger in order to perceive the thickening of the superior border of the bone.

*Comment:* **In this photograph, the digital grip is positioned facing the investigated structure, which is palpated by the index finger.**

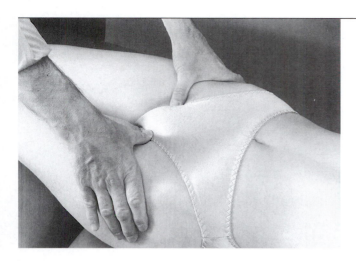

## FIGURE 1-7
### THE PUBIC TUBERCLE

With your hands laid flat at the level of the greater trochanter bilaterally, your thumbs move horizontally and medially, searching across the pubic region (the mons veneris) for a spine-shaped bony prominence (the pubic tubercle). This is located over the most medial part of the horizontal ramus of the pubis, next to the symphysis pubis and more precisely at the junction of the "pectineal crest" and the anterior lip of the "subpubic groove."

*Comment:*     ***In male subjects, be careful with the spermatic cord during this examination.***

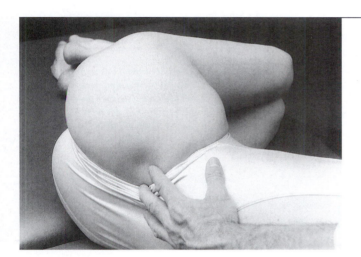

## FIGURE 1-8
### THE POSTEROSUPERIOR ILIAC SPINE

This structure, which faces the sacroiliac joint, corresponds to a more or less visible dimple.

It can also be demonstrated by finding the most posterior segment of the iliac crest and following it to its junction with the posterior border of the iliac bone. The latter is characterized by a slight depression representing the small "coxal notch."

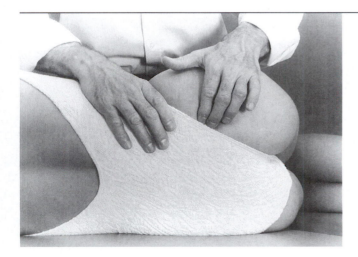

## FIGURE 1-9
### THE SMALL "COXAL NOTCH" AND
### THE POSTEROINFERIOR ILIAC SPINE

#### THE SMALL COXAL NOTCH

The small coxal notch is located between the posterosuperior iliac spine and the posteroinferior iliac spine at approximately two finger breadths from the latter. By moving the pelvis forward and back, this structure is more easily found.

#### THE POSTEROINFERIOR ILIAC SPINE

A bidigital grip, positioned approximately two fingerbreadths from the posterosuperior iliac spine, determines its localization. It is better perceived when the pelvis is alternately moved forward and back.

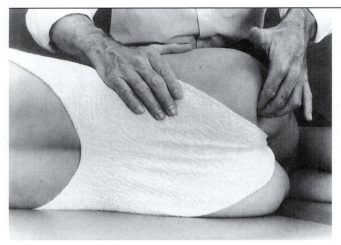

**FIGURE 1-10**
**THE ISCHIAL SPINE AND THE LESSER SCIATIC NOTCH**

## THE ISCHIAL SPINE

With the subject lying on his or her side and the hip in flexion, locate the ischial tuberosity and move upward to the lesser sciatic notch, using a digital grip.

Then, apply your grip against the ischial tuberosity and slide it into the lesser sciatic notch without losing the pressure point on the skin (by this maneuver, the skin will slide on top of the underlying tissues). The ischial spine is located at the proximal end of this notch.

*Comment:*     *The gluteus maximus muscle must be relaxed.*

## THE LESSER SCIATIC NOTCH

The ischial tuberosity must first be located using a bidigital grip (see Fig. 1-12).

The depression palpated above the tuberosity, towards the sacrum, is the lesser sciatic notch.

*Comment:*     *This structure is located between the ischial spine and the ischial tuberosity. The gluteus maximus muscle must be relaxed. It is sometimes preferable to leave the hip in a much less flexed position than shown in this picture. This allows better penetration of the grip through the mass of the gluteal muscle, which becomes less tense.*

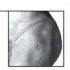

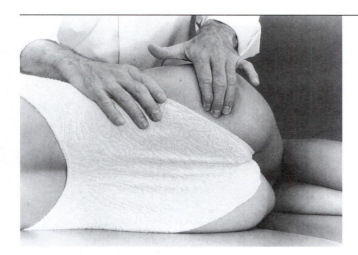

## FIGURE 1-11
### THE GREATER SCIATIC NOTCH

First locate the posteroinferior iliac spine using bidigital palpation. Lean on the external structure of the ilium. Then move your grip backward towards the greater ischial notch and the lateral border of the sacrum.

*Comment:*   *This structure, wide and deep, is located between the posteroinferior iliac spine and the ischial spine. It is examined through the muscular mass of the gluteus maximus muscle and is therefore difficult to access.*

*Keep in mind that its concavity is posterior and that the piriformis muscle as well as the great ischial nerve pass through it. The examination must be carried out accordingly.*

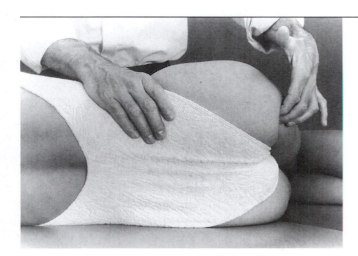

## FIGURE 1-12
### THE ISCHIAL TUBEROSITY

This structure is oval in shape with a large posterosuperior end; its narrow inferior end extends from the inferior border of the iliac bone. Flexion of the hip clears it from the gluteus maximus muscle.

It is also possible to palpate this structure with the subject prone. It is then found in the middle of the cutaneous landmark formed by the gluteal fold.

*Comment:*   *Most of the time, in sitting, one sits on the ischial tuberosities.*

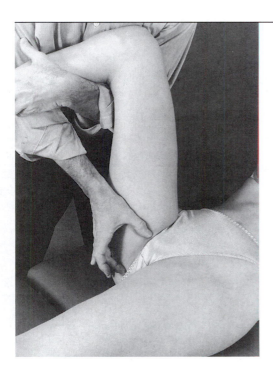

## FIGURE 1-13
### THE INFERIOR BORDER OF THE ILIAC BONE

Locate the ischial tuberosity (Fig. 1-12) and the most anterior and medial part of the descending ramus of the pubis.

The inferior border of the iliac bone is easily accessible between these two bony structures.

# THE FEMUR

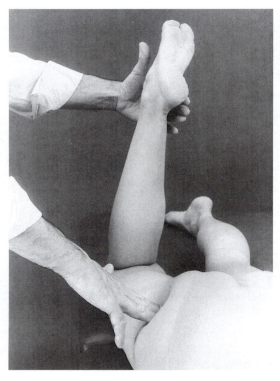

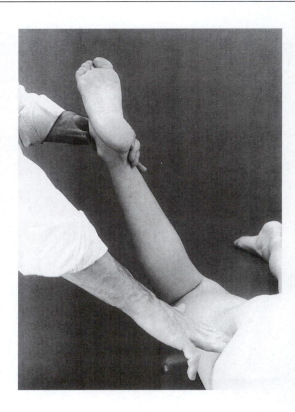

**FIGURES 1-14 AND 1-15**
**POSTERIOR APPROACH TO THE FEMORAL HEAD**

The hip is mobilized by rotating it medially in order to push the femoral head posteriorly. The head is accessible through the muscular mass of the gluteus maximus between the greater trochanter and the lateral surface of the iliac bone.

For improved palpation of the head beneath your fingers, rotate the hip several times.

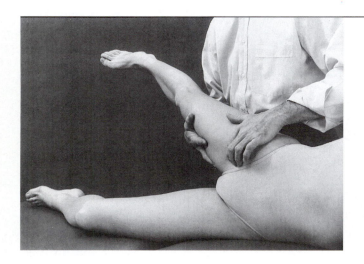

**FIGURE 1-16**
**ANTERIOR APPROACH TO THE FEMORAL HEAD**

With the subject lying on his or her side, stand behind the subject and stabilize the pelvis with your hip (in the anteroposterior plane).

Place your proximal hand on the anterolateral aspect of the hip and grip its anterior aspect, using your finger and thumb.

Your distal hand supports the anteromedial aspect of the thigh as you slowly bring the limb into extension (stabilizing the pelvis with your hip).

The fingers of your proximal hand will gradually perceive the femoral head, which is a density projecting forward.

*Comment:*   *During this mobilization, you can perceive the pulse of the femoral artery, which is pushed forward by the femoral head.*

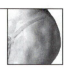

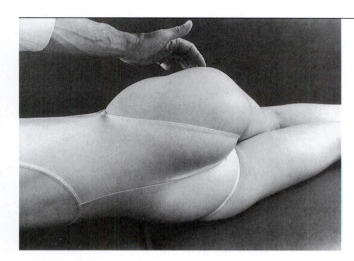

## FIGURE 1-17
### APPROACH TO THE GREATER TROCHANTER WITH THE SUBJECT LYING ON HIS OR HER SIDE

In this position, the greater trochanter projects on the lateral aspect of the hip.

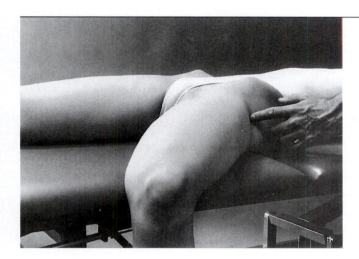

## FIGURE 1-18
### APPROACH TO THE GREATER TROCHANTER WITH THE SUBJECT SUPINE

In the supine position, with the lower extremity in slight abduction, the greater trochanter is accessible in the skin depression created by the hip abduction. This position also allows optimal relaxation of the surrounding muscles, facilitating access to the different parts of the greater trochanter, including the superior border, inferior border, anterior border, posterior border, and lateral surface.

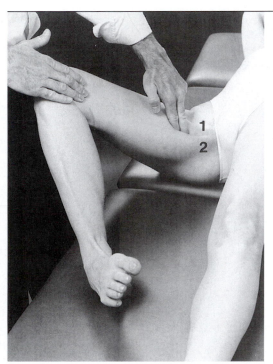

**FIGURE 1-19**

**THE LESSER TROCHANTER. STEP 1: DEMONSTRATE THE DEPRESSION BETWEEN THE ADDUCTOR LONGUS MUSCLE (1) AND THE GRACILIS MUSCLE (2)**

In this figure, you can see the gracilis muscle (2) in a posteromedial position.

With the subject supine, the hip and knee are flexed. As you proceed, you must resist a movement of adduction. The goal of this technique is to demonstrate these two muscular structures, between which you can make direct contact with the lesser trochanter.

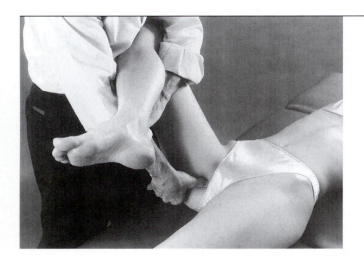

**FIGURE 1-20**

**THE LESSER TROCHANTER. STEP 2: MAKE DIRECT CONTACT**

The dorsal aspect of your one hand supports the lateral aspect of the leg and allows a forward movement of the lesser trochanter through an external rotation of the hip. The thumb of your other hand then slides through the soft tissues between the adductor longus and gracilis muscles, looking for a somewhat sensitive density.

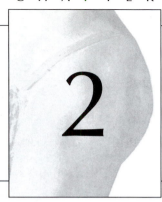

# 2

# MYOLOGY

## THE LATERAL INGUINOFEMORAL REGION

Triangular in shape with its apex proximal, this region is defined by

- the apex (proximal), formed by the anterosuperior iliac spine
- the lateral border, formed by the tensor fascia lata muscle (Fig. 2-2)
- the medial border, formed by the sartorius muscle (Fig. 2-4)

- the floor of this triangular space, formed by the rectus femoris muscle (Fig. 2-3), the proximal end of which infiltrates between the two muscles mentioned above

*Comment:* **The muscles delineating this region belong to the topographic region of the thigh.**

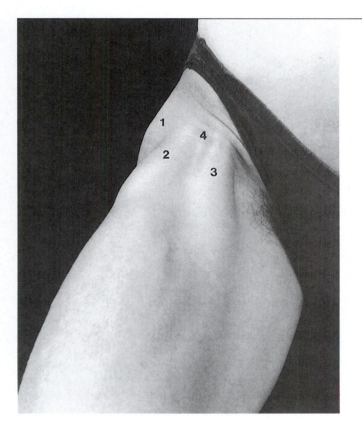

**FIGURE 2-1**
**ANTEROMEDIAL VIEW**

1. Gluteus medius muscle
2. Tensor muscle of the fascia lata
3. Sartorius muscle
4. Rectus femoris muscle

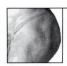

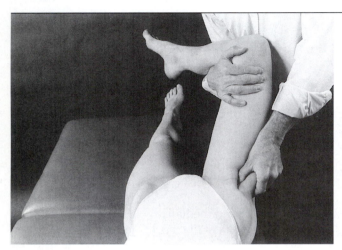

### FIGURE 2-2
#### TENSOR MUSCLE OF THE FASCIA LATA

A resistance placed against the anteromedial aspect of the thigh in flexion demonstrates two muscles in the proximal part of the thigh. The most lateral one is the tensor fascia lata.

This muscle is located between the anterosuperior iliac spine and the greater trochanter.

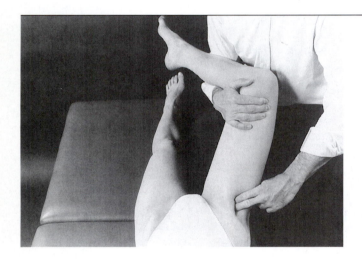

### FIGURE 2-3
#### THE RECTUS FEMORIS MUSCLE

The most proximal portion of this muscle is found in the depression between the tensor muscle of the fascia lata laterally and the sartorius muscle medially.

Even in its relaxed state, the proximal aspect of this muscle can be palpated easily. If you request an extension of the knee, the muscular fibers will be more readily palpable.

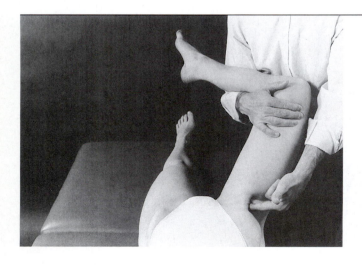

### FIGURE 2-4
#### THE SARTORIUS MUSCLE

The technique here is similar to that used to palpate the tensor muscle of the fascia lata. The sartorius muscle corresponds to the most medial muscle mass demonstrated in the proximal portion of the thigh. The anterosuperior iliac spine is the bony landmark, since this muscle originates from it.

*Comment:*     ***The sartorius muscle forms the medial border of the lateral inguinofemoral region. It is also the lateral border of the medial inguinofemoral region or femoral triangle.***

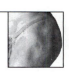

# THE MEDIAL INGUINOFEMORAL REGION OR FEMORAL TRIANGLE

Triangular in shape with an inferior apex, this region, called Scarpa's triangle, is delimited by

- the base (proximal), formed by the inguinal ligament; it joins the anterosuperior iliac spine and the pubic tubercle
- the lateral border, formed by the sartorius muscle (Fig. 2-4)
- the medial border, formed by the adductor longus muscle (Fig. 2-6)

- the apex (distal) (Fig. 2-5), formed by the junction between the sartorius and the adductor longus muscles (Fig. 2-6)
- the floor, formed medially by the pectineus muscles (Fig. 2-7) and laterally by the iliopsoas muscle (Fig. 2-8). This muscular mass forms a concave groove in which the neurovascular bundle of the lower limb lies

*Comment:*    *The sartorius, adductor longus, and pectineus muscles belong to the thigh region.*

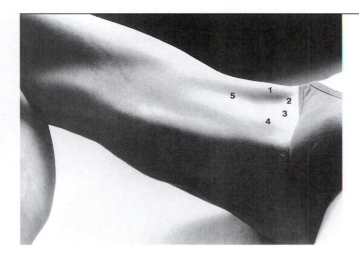

**FIGURE 2-5**
**MEDIAL VIEW**

1. Sartorius muscle
2. Iliopsoas muscle
3. Pectineus muscle
4. Adductor longus muscle
5. Apex of Scarpa's triangle, the junction point between the sartorius and adductor longus muscles

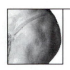

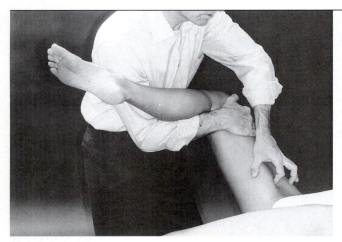

### FIGURE 2-6
#### THE ADDUCTOR LONGUS MUSCLE

With the hip and knee in flexion, the lower extremity is abducted and your hand supports the lower thigh. Resistance against a movement of adduction demonstrates the adductor longus muscle, which appears at the superomedial aspect of the thigh.

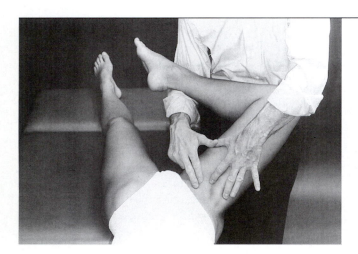

### FIGURE 2-7
#### THE PECTINEUS MUSCLE

This muscle is found in the depression just lateral to the adductor longus muscle. It forms the medial aspect of the floor of Scarpa's triangle.

In this figure, the sartorius muscle is shown between the index and the middle fingers of the left hand (resisting the flexion and the adduction of the hip). The other hand shows the pectineus muscle.

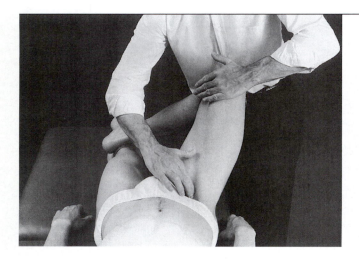

### FIGURE 2-8
#### THE ILIOPSOAS MUSCLE IN ITS DISTAL ASPECT

Your grip must be placed medial to the proximal course of the sartorius muscle, close to its insertion on the anterosuperior iliac spine. The iliopsoas muscle is accessible at this level since it reflects on the iliopectineal surface, covering, beyond this reflection, the anterior aspect of the femoral joint. It is lined medially by the pectineus muscle. When it is placed under tension (as you resist hip flexion with your distal hand), you can palpate this muscle's contracting fibers at the level of the "iliopectineal process."

*Comment:     This region is sensitive and should be approached with care.*

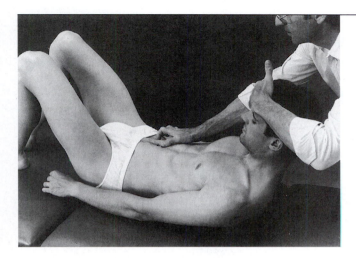

### Figure 2-9
### The iliopsoas muscle in its proximal portion.
### Step 1: Find the landmarks

Resistance placed against the subject's forehead allows the abdominal muscles and therefore the lateral border of the rectus abdominis muscle to protrude. Your thumb is placed on the umbilicus and the middle finger on the anterosuperior iliac spine. Your index finger is placed in the midportion of this line, at the lateral border of the rectus abdominis muscle.

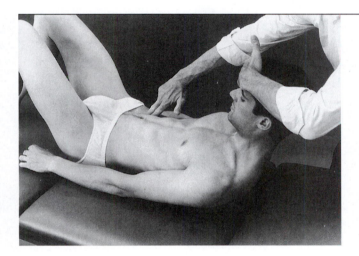

### Figure 2-10
### The iliopsoas muscle in its proximal portion. Step 2

The lateral border of the rectus abdominis muscle, as shown, is the optimal point at which to approach the iliopsoas muscle.

The subject's head is allowed to lie on a pillow in order to relax the abdominal muscles. You may change position and stand at the level of the subject's hip in order to pursue the examination. It is essential to examine the abdominal muscles with caution and in a stepwise fashion in order to prevent guarding of the abdominal wall.

By actively flexing the subject's hip, you will create muscular tension and obtain a better idea of the structures examined.

*Comment:*     *This figure demonstrates the starting point for the examination and not the technique of palpation.*

# THE GLUTEAL REGION

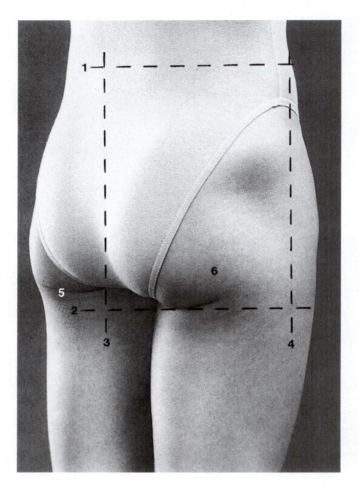

**FIGURE 2-11**
**POSTEROLATERAL VIEW**

1. Superior border: iliac crest
2. Inferior border: gluteal fold
3. Medial border: iliac crest and, following, the coccyx
4. Lateral border: this is an imaginary vertical line starting at the anterosuperior iliac spine and extending downward to the level of the greater trochanter, where it joins the lateralmost aspect of the gluteal fold or its continuation

*Comment:*    *This imaginary line is noteworthy as it lines up more or less with the posterior border of the tensor muscle of the fascia lata.*

5. Gluteal fold
6. Gluteus maximus muscle

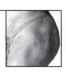

# SUPERFICIAL PLANE

The superficial plane of the gluteal region is represented by a single muscle: the gluteus maximus (Fig. 2-13).

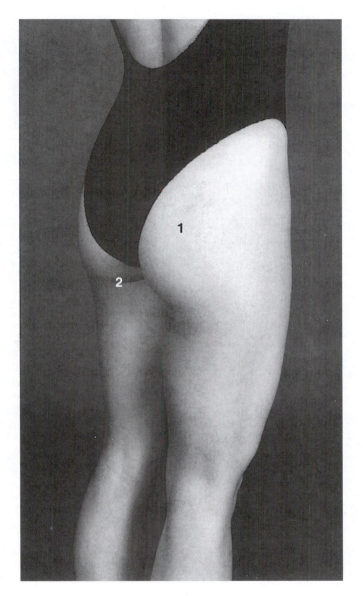

**FIGURE 2-12**
**THE GLUTEUS MAXIMUS MUSCLE**

Posterolateral view
1. Gluteus maximus muscle
2. Gluteal fold

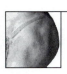

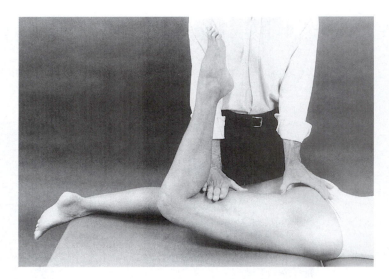

### FIGURE 2-13
### THE GLUTEUS MAXIMUS MUSCLE

The technique demonstrated above allows visualization of the gluteus maximus muscle.

The iliac crest, the greater trochanter, and the ischial tuberosity are the essential bony landmarks surrounding the gluteal region.

The gluteal fold, which has an essentially horizontal course, corresponds approximately with the inferior border of this muscle, which follows an oblique course downward and laterally.

The subject is asked to lift the anterior aspect of the thigh off the table, keeping the knee flexed and without any compensation at the level of the lumbar region. Place resistance against the inferoposterior aspect of the thigh to prevent prompting of the knee, allowing the muscular mass to project and demonstrate the quality of the contraction as compared with that of the contralateral muscle.

*Comment:* **The flexion of the knee, by shortening the hamstring muscles, favors the activity of the gluteus maximus muscle (i.e., extension of the hip).**

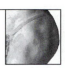

# MIDDLE PLANE

The middle plane of the gluteal region is represented by a single muscle: the gluteus medius (Figs. 2-15 and 2-16).

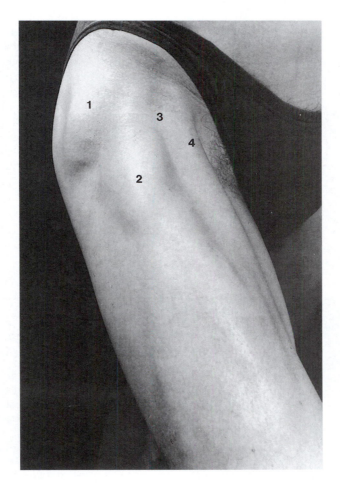

**FIGURE 2-14**
**ANTEROLATERAL VIEW OF THE HIP**

1.  Gluteus medius muscle
2.  Tensor muscle of the fascia lata
3.  Rectus femoris muscle
4.  Sartorius muscle

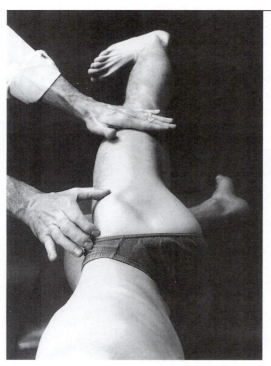

### FIGURE 2-15
### THE GLUTEUS MEDIUS MUSCLE

The essential bony landmarks are the anterior part of the iliac crest and the superior border of the greater trochanter.

Place your hands as illustrated and ask the subject to abduct against resistance; the muscular body will tighten between your fingers.

With the hip in abduction, ask the subject to perform rapid, consecutive internal rotations of the hip in order to mobilize the anterior fibers of the gluteus medius muscle more specifically. This movement also mobilizes the gluteus minimus muscle. In any event, this additional movement improves digital perception of the muscular body.

*Comment:*   *The hand creating the resistance should be placed against the lateral and inferior portion of the thigh, just above the knee (in order to prevent prompting of the knee).*

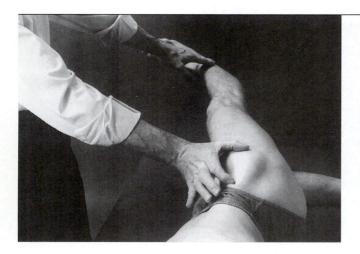

### FIGURE 2-16
### TECHNIQUE TO DISTINGUISH THE GLUTEUS MEDIUS MUSCLE FROM THE TENSOR MUSCLE OF THE FASCIA LATA

From the same position, the subject should be asked to flex the hip slightly (with some guidance), keeping it in abduction, so that you may demonstrate the muscular body of the tensor muscle of the fascia lata between your fingers.

*Comment:*   *The vertical imaginary line drawn from the anterosuperior iliac spine to the greater trochanter, which delimits the gluteal region (Fig. 2-11) anteriorly, represents the posterior border of the tensor muscle of the fascia lata, which extends inferiorly onto the anterior part of the thigh (see also Fig. 2-14).*

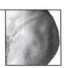

# DEEP PLANE

The deep plane of the gluteal region includes the following:

- the gluteus minimus muscle (Fig. 2-18)
- the piriformis muscle (Figs. 2-19 through 2-22)
- the inferior and superior gemellus muscles (Fig. 2-23)
- the obturator medialis muscle (Fig. 2-23)
- the quadratus femoris muscle (Fig. 2-24)
- the obturator lateralis muscle (Fig. 2-25)

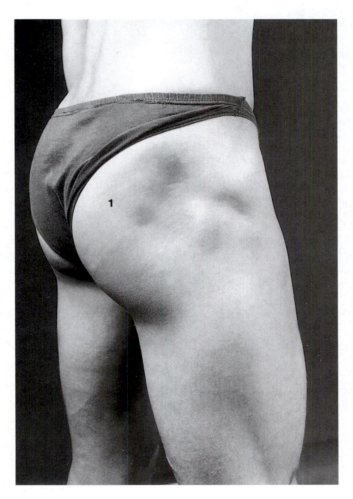

**FIGURE 2-17**
**POSTEROLATERAL VIEW OF THE HIP**

*Comment:*    **The gluteus minimus muscle can be approached only through the muscular body of the gluteus medius muscle (Fig. 2-14). The other muscles of the deep plane can be approached only through the gluteus maximus muscle (1) (Fig. 2-17).**

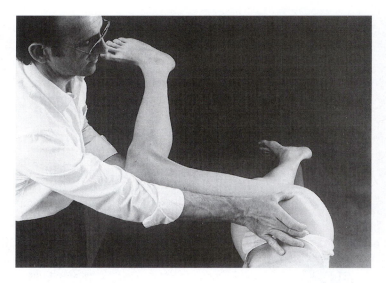

**FIGURE 2-18**
**THE GLUTEUS MINIMUS MUSCLE**

Place your proximal palpating hand between the superior border of the greater trochanter and the most anterior part of the iliac crest, between the tubercle of the gluteus medius muscle and the antero-superior iliac spine.

In this position, your thumb, opposed by the other fingers of your hand, straddles the gluteus minimus muscle, which is located under the gluteus medius muscle. Your distal hand supports the medial aspect of the knee and leg.

From this original position (hip and knee flexed at 90°), the subject is asked to perform an internal rotation of the hip. Practically speaking, the leg will be mobilized upward. A muscular mass corresponding to the gluteus medius and gluteus minimus muscles will move beneath your fingers.

*Comment:* *Only the muscle's contraction is perceptible beneath your fingers. Direct access to the muscle is not possible, since it is covered by the anterior fibers of the gluteus medius muscle, which have the same actions as those of the gluteus minimus muscle.*

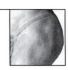

**The piriformis muscle is approached in four steps:**

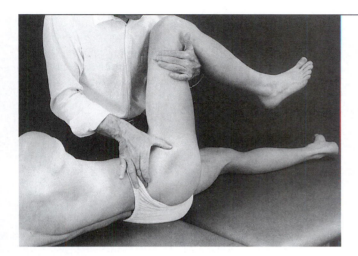

### FIGURE 2-19
### STEP 1: LOCATE THE GLUTEUS MEDIUS MUSCLE AND THE DEPRESSION AT THE BOTTOM OF IT, FROM WHICH THE PIRIFORMIS MUSCLE IS APPROACHED

The subject is placed on his or her side. With one supporting hand, bring the limb to be examined against your shoulder or chest. From this position, ask the subject to abduct against resistance horizontally. This muscular action allows the gluteus medius muscle to protrude.

*Comment:*    *Interestingly, this step demonstrates both the posterior border of this muscle as well as the depression that follows posteriorly, at the bottom of which is the piriformis muscle.*

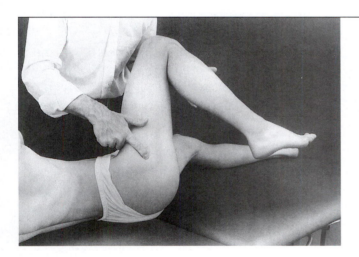

### FIGURE 2-20
### STEP 2: LOCATE THE GREATER TROCHANTER

The subject is placed on his or her side. With the subject's knee flexed, your distal hand grabs the medial aspect of the leg and knee in order to mobilize the hip in all planes, thereby demonstrating the greater trochanter. Refer also to Chap. 1, "Osteology," for more details about this structure.

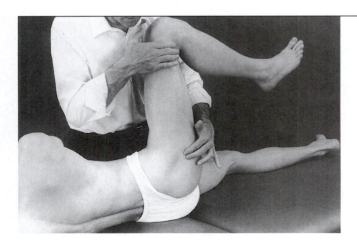

### FIGURE 2-21
### STEP 3: LOCATE THE SUPEROLATERAL BORDER OF THE GREATER TROCHANTER, THE INSERTION POINT OF THE PIRIFORMIS MUSCLE

While your one hand resists a horizontal abduction of the hip, your other hand is placed in the distal part of the demonstrated depression, in contact with the greater trochanter.

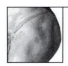

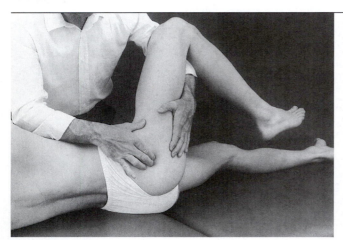

### FIGURE 2-22
### THE PIRIFORMIS MUSCLE

The subject's hip is flexed at 45° and the knee at 90°. Your proximal hand is placed on the upper part of the posterior border of the greater trochanter, at its junction with the superior border and in contact with the posterior border of the gluteus medius muscle. To appreciate the latter, ask the subject to rotate the hip internally or abduct it horizontally. Better yet, these two movements can be combined or alternated. A depression originating from the posterosuperior angle of the greater trochanter and extending toward the iliac crest will take shape under the skin and indicate the posterior border of the gluteus medius muscle through the anterior fibers of the gluteus maximus muscle.

The limb should be palpated through a perfectly relaxed gluteus maximus muscle, toward the greater sciatic notch and the lateral border of the sacrum, by following the posterior border of the gluteus medius muscle, as demonstrated previously.

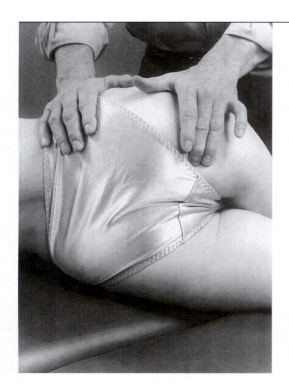

### FIGURE 2-23
### THE INFERIOR AND SUPERIOR GEMELLUS MUSCLES AND THE OBTURATOR MEDIALIS MUSCLE

A bidigital grip at the level of the lesser sciatic notch makes it possible to palpate these muscles through the mass of the gluteus maximus muscle.

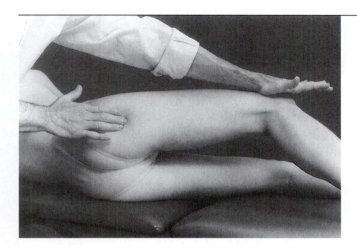

## FIGURE 2-24
### THE QUADRATUS FEMORIS MUSCLE

Direct examination of this muscle is not possible, since it is located under the gluteus maximus muscle.

The essential bony landmarks are the ischial tuberosity medially and the greater trochanter laterally.

The essential muscular landmark is the inferior border of the gluteus maximus muscle.

With the subject lying on his or her side and the hip slightly flexed, resistance is applied to the lateral aspect of the knee against an external rotation and abduction of the hip. The body of the muscle will tighten beneath your fingers through the mass of the gluteus maximus muscle (which should be perfectly relaxed) over its inferior aspect and between the bony landmarks described previously. The palpation is difficult in the normal subject.

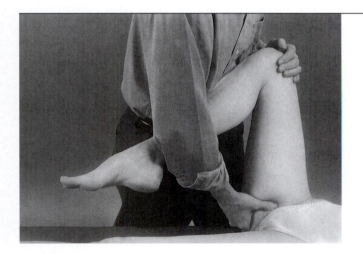

## FIGURE 2-25
### THE OBTURATOR LATERALIS MUSCLE

The subject's knee and hip are flexed at 90°. The thumb of your palpating hand is placed between the adductor longus and gracilis muscles (see Fig. 1-19). Your right arm applies resistance against an external rotation of the hip while you ask the subject to perform a sequence of contractions and relaxations. This muscular action tenses the muscle of interest, as perceived beneath your thumb. The other hand also supports the limb.

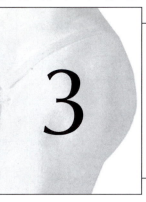

C H A P T E R

# 3

# NERVES AND VESSELS

## THE MEDIAL INGUINOFEMORAL REGION OR SCARPA'S TRIANGLE

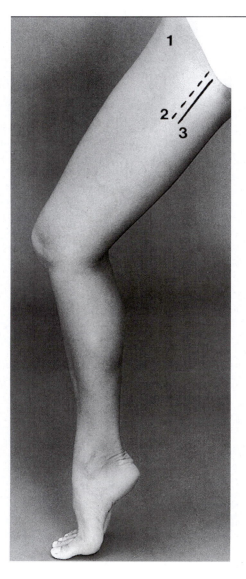

**FIGURE 3-1**
**MEDIAL VIEW OF THE THIGH**

1.  Sartorius muscle
2.  Femoral nerve
3.  Femoral artery

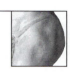

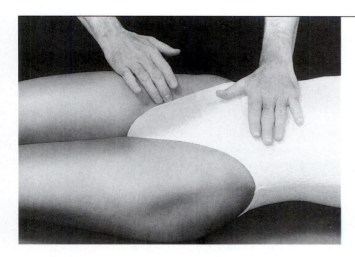

## FIGURE 3-2
### THE FEMORAL ARTERY

Perform a bidigital palpation with slight compression along the artery, in the middle of an imaginary line drawn between the anterosuperior iliac spine and the pubic tubercle. The arterial pulse will be better perceived with the hip in a neutral position or slight extension.

*Note:* Over the medial aspect of the artery, you may perceive superficial small round structures. These represent superficial inguinal lymph nodes.

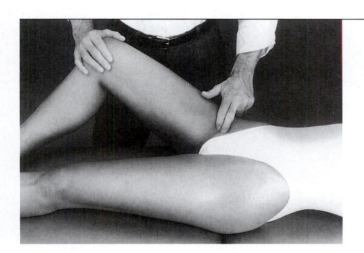

## FIGURE 3-3
### THE FEMORAL NERVE: STEP 1

As for the examination of the femoral pulse (Figure 1-47), the first maneuver is to perform a bidigital palpation in the middle of an imaginary line drawn between the anterosuperior iliac spine and the pubic tubercle.

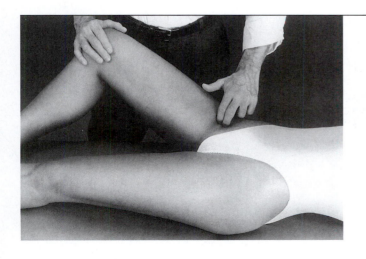

## FIGURE 3-4
### THE FEMORAL NERVE: STEP 2

In this step, your grip should be moved laterally by one fingerbreadth toward the sartorius muscle so that it is positioned on top of the investigated structure. This should be approached carefully with a digital "claw type" grip, as shown in the figure, and with the caution required for this type of structure. The nerve is palpated beneath your fingers as a full cylindrical cord.

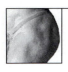

# THE GLUTEAL REGION

# THE GREATER SCIATIC NERVE

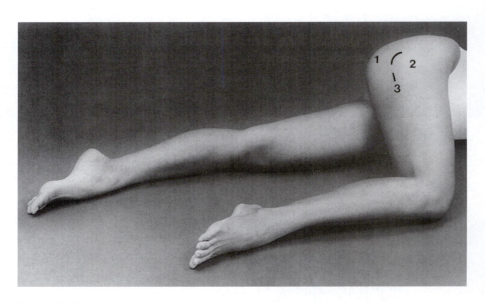

**FIGURE 3-5**
**LATERAL VIEW OF THE GLUTEAL REGION**

1. Ischial tuberosity
2. Greater trochanter
3. Sciatic nerve

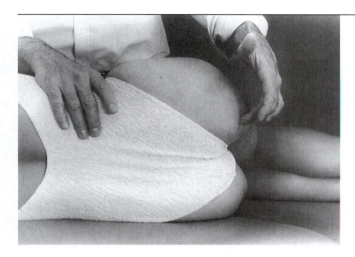

### FIGURE 3-6
#### LOCATING THE GREATER SCIATIC NERVE. STEP 1: DEMONSTRATE THE ISCHIAL TUBEROSITY

In this position, where the hip is flexed, the ischial tuberosity is normally cleared from the gluteus maximus muscle. A bidigital grip (middle and ring fingers) should be placed over it.

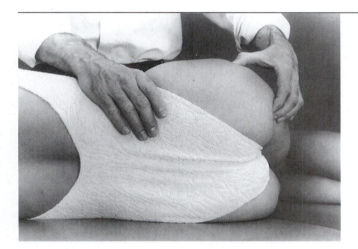

### FIGURE 3-7
#### LOCATING THE GREATER SCIATIC NERVE. STEP 2: DEMONSTRATE THE GREATER TROCHANTER

While you maintain the previous grip (Fig. 3-6), your thumb is positioned over the greater trochanter.

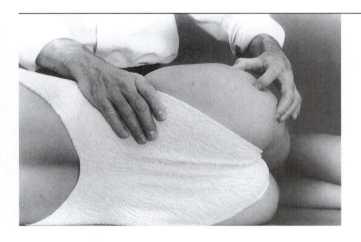

### FIGURE 3-8
#### LOCATING THE GREATER SCIATIC NERVE. STEP 3

Imagine a line drawn between the two demonstrated bony structures. Place your index finger approximately in the middle. This is where the greater sciatic nerve normally lies.

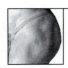

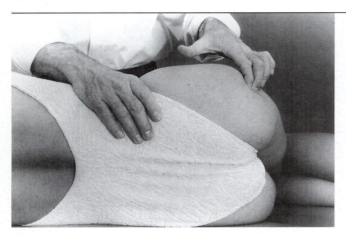

**FIGURE 3-9**
**THE GREATER SCIATIC NERVE. STEP 4**

At this level, the nerve's diameter is approximately one fingerbreadth. It should be approached transversely and cautiously with a bidigital grip.

*Comment:* *The nerve is accessible only if the subject's morphology will allow for it and only through a perfectly relaxed gluteus maximus muscle. In that case, a full cylindrical cord is palpated under the fingers.*

# THE
# THIGH

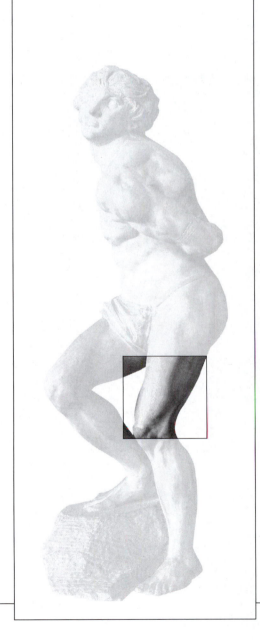

## ILLUSTRATED STUDY OF THE THIGH (ANTERIOR)

## ILLUSTRATED STUDY OF THE THIGH (POSTERIOR)

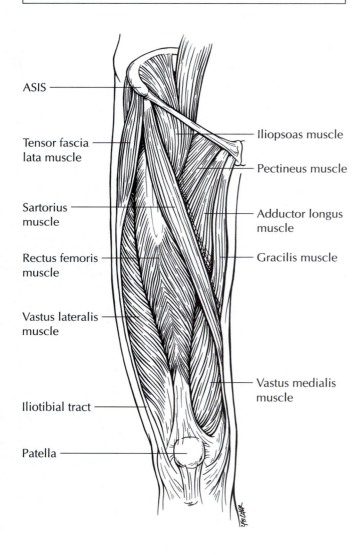

ASIS

Tensor fascia lata muscle

Sartorius muscle

Rectus femoris muscle

Vastus lateralis muscle

Iliotibial tract

Patella

Iliopsoas muscle

Pectineus muscle

Adductor longus muscle

Gracilis muscle

Vastus medialis muscle

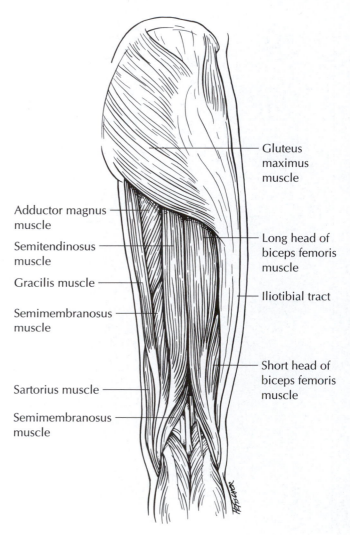

Gluteus maximus muscle

Adductor magnus muscle

Semitendinosus muscle

Gracilis muscle

Semimembranosus muscle

Sartorius muscle

Semimembranosus muscle

Long head of biceps femoris muscle

Iliotibial tract

Short head of biceps femoris muscle

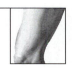

# ILLUSTRATED STUDY OF THE THIGH (LATERAL)

# ILLUSTRATED STUDY OF THE THIGH (MEDIAL)

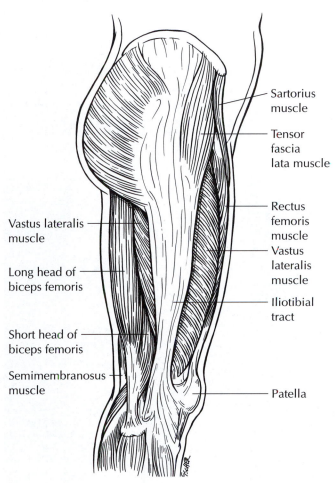

Sartorius muscle

Tensor fascia lata muscle

Rectus femoris muscle

Vastus lateralis muscle

Iliotibial tract

Patella

Vastus lateralis muscle

Long head of biceps femoris

Short head of biceps femoris

Semimembranosus muscle

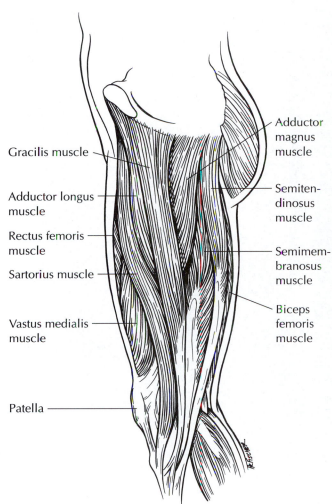

Gracilis muscle

Adductor longus muscle

Rectus femoris muscle

Sartorius muscle

Vastus medialis muscle

Patella

Adductor magnus muscle

Semitendinosus muscle

Semimembranosus muscle

Biceps femoris muscle

# TOPOGRAPHIC PRESENTATION OF THE THIGH (FEMUR)

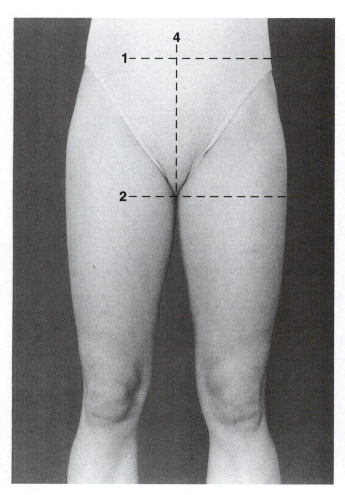

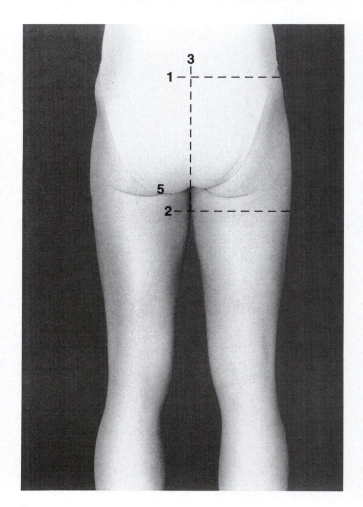

**FIGURE 4-1**
**ANTERIOR VIEW**

1.  Superior border

**FIGURE 4-2**
**POSTERIOR VIEW**

2.  Inferior border

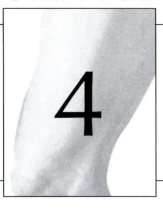

# 4

# MYOLOGY

# THE ANTEROFEMORAL REGION:
# THE ANTERIOR MUSCULAR GROUP

This region is formed by the anterior muscular group, which includes the following:

- the sartorius muscle (Figs. 4-5, 4-6, and 4-7)
- the quadriceps extensor muscle, which includes:
  —the vastus medialis muscle (Fig. 4-10)
  —the vastus lateralis muscle (Fig. 4-11)
  —the rectus femoris muscle (Figs. 4-12 and 4-13)
  —the vastus intermedius muscle, which is not discussed in this book
- the tensor muscle of the fascia lata and the iliotibial tract (Figs. 4-15, 4-16, and 4-17)

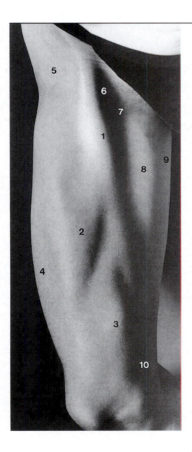

**FIGURE 4-3**
**ANTEROMEDIAL VIEW OF THE THIGH**

1. Sartorius muscle
2. Rectus femoris muscle
3. Vastus medialis muscle
4. Vastus lateralis muscle
5. Tensor muscle of the fascia lata
6. Iliopsoas muscle
7. Pectineus muscle
8. Adductor longus muscle
9. Gracilis muscle
10. Distal tendon of insertion of the adductor magnus muscle: insertion into the adductor tubercle on the medial condyle of the femur

# THE SARTORIUS MUSCLE

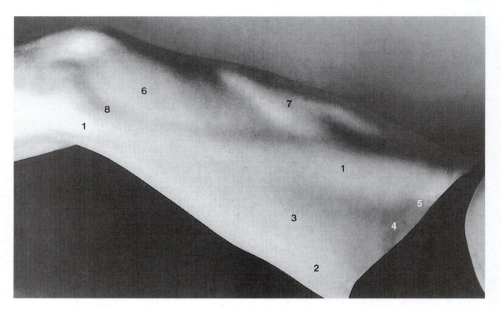

**FIGURE 4-4**
**MEDIAL VIEW OF THE SARTORIUS MUSCLE AND DEMONSTRATION OF ITS RELATIONSHIPS WITH THE OTHER THIGH MUSCLES**

1. Sartorius muscle
2. Gracilis muscle
3. Adductor longus muscle
4. Pectineus muscle
5. Iliopsoas muscle
6. Vastus medialis muscle
7. Rectus femoris muscle
8. Distal tendon of insertion of the adductor magnus muscle: insertion into the adductor tubercle on the medial condyle of the femur

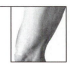

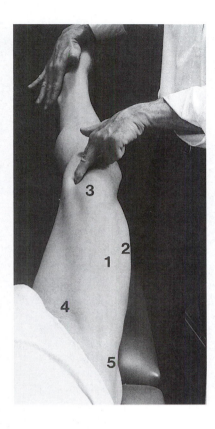

## FIGURE 4-5

### THE SARTORIUS MUSCLE IN ITS DISTAL ASPECT

Ask the subject to maintain an almost complete isometric extension of the knee and a slight flexion of the hip.

In order to resist its adduction isometrically, the hip should be rotated externally and a resistance should be applied on the inferomedial aspect of the leg.

*Comment:*     ***The proximal hand pulls the sartorius muscle away from the vastus medialis muscle (3).***

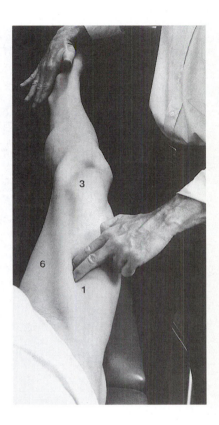

## FIGURE 4-6 ➡

### THE SARTORIUS MUSCLE AT THE THIGH LEVEL

The technique of placing the muscle under tension is the same as that described above. When it is not under tension, it is a flat muscle, which creates a depression at the junction of the anterior and medial compartments of the thigh. The adductor muscles adjoin its medial aspect, while the vastus medialis muscle (3) distally and the rectus femoris muscle (1) proximally adjoin its lateral aspect.

---

### FIGURES 4-5, 4-6, AND 4-7

1.   Rectus femoris muscle
2.   Vastus lateralis muscle
3.   Vastus medialis muscle
4.   Pectineus muscle
5.   Tensor muscle of the fascia lata
6.   Adductor muscles

---

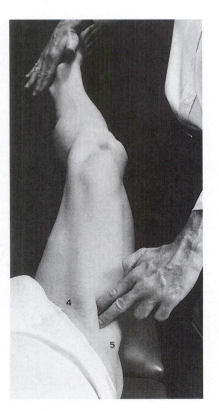

## FIGURE 4-7

### THE SARTORIUS MUSCLE IN ITS PROXIMAL ASPECT

The technique of putting the muscle under tension is the same as that described in Fig. 4-5.

The proximal portion appears near the anterosuperior iliac spine (see also the region of the hip).

To push the sartorius muscle medially, position your grip in the depression between the sartorius muscle and the tensor muscle of the fascia lata (5). The iliopsoas muscle, not shown in this picture, and the pectineus muscle (4) adjoin its medial aspect.

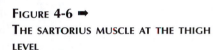

# THE QUADRICEPS EXTENSOR MUSCLE

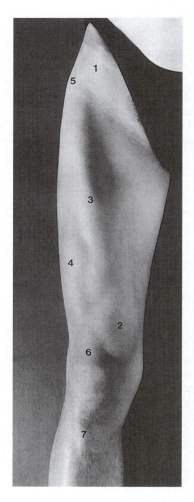

**FIGURE 4-8**
**ANTERIOR VIEW OF THE THIGH**

1. Sartorius muscle
2. Vastus medialis muscle
3. Rectus femoris muscle
4. Vastus lateralis muscle
5. Tensor muscle of the fascia lata
6. Tendon of the quadriceps extensor muscle
7. Patellar ligament

*Comment:* **The crureus muscle, which forms the deep portion of the quadriceps extensor muscle, is not visible.**

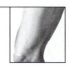

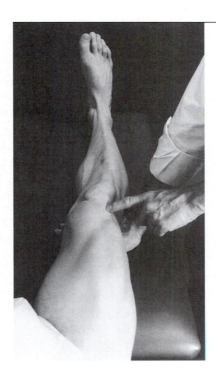

### FIGURE 4-9
#### THE TENDON OF THE QUADRICEPS EXTENSOR MUSCLE

Your distal hand is placed under the knee to ensure that the contraction is performed properly. The subject is asked to carry out sequences of contraction-relaxation of the quadriceps extensor muscle. Note that your hand should be pressed against the table. The examination of the tendon proceeds above the level of the patella and between the vastus medialis and vastus lateralis muscles (figure below).

*Comment:*     *For the patellar ligament, see Fig. 6-15 on page 80 in Part III, "The Knee."*

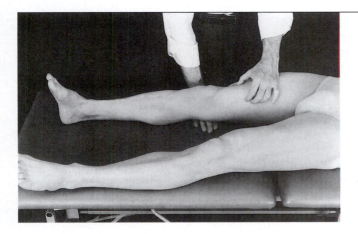

### FIGURE 4-10
#### THE VASTUS MEDIALIS MUSCLE

To demonstrate this muscle, the subject must perform a knee extension. With the dorsum of your hand under the subject's knee at the level of the popliteal fossa, ask the subject to press your hand against the table. Your other hand palpates the vastus medialis muscle, which appears over the inferomedial aspect of the thigh.

*Comment:*     *The topographic characteristic of the vastus medialis muscle is that its distal end extends more distally than that of the vastus lateralis muscle (approximately four fingerbreadths).*

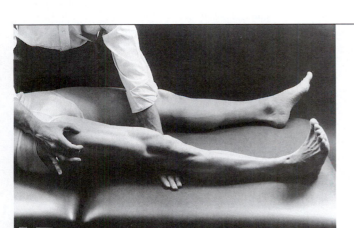

### FIGURE 4-11
#### THE VASTUS LATERALIS MUSCLE

This muscle is located over the lateral surface of the thigh, lateral to the vastus intermedius muscle; its lateral surface is covered by the iliotibial tract or Maissiat's band (see Figs. 4-15 and 4-16).

The technique to put the muscle under tension is the same as that described for the vastus medialis muscle (Fig. 4-10).

*Comment:*     *Remember that this muscle extends posteriorly slightly beyond the iliotibial tract or Maissiat's band.*

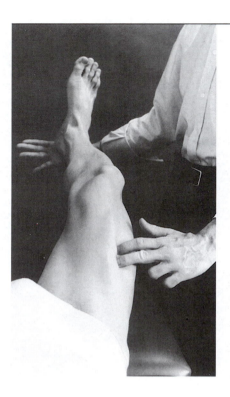

## Figure 4-12
### The rectus femoris muscle at the thigh level

The hip is in slight flexion and the knee in partial extension. Your hand is placed under the heel in order to modulate this position. Ask the subject to maintain an isometric contraction of the quadriceps extensor muscle.

In most subjects, this muscle appears over the medial aspect of the thigh between the vastus medialis muscle medially and the vastus lateralis muscle laterally. In the others, one must look for the muscular mass in contraction through a varying thickness of adipose tissue.

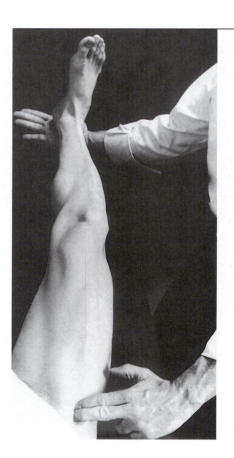

## Figure 4-13
### The rectus femoris muscle in its proximal portion

The hip is flexed and the knee is in partial extension in order to demonstrate the muscular body.

Your distal hand is placed under the subject's heel in order to control the requested movements.

Ask the subject to lift the heel slightly off your supporting hand, creating a contraction of the muscular body between the sartorius muscle medially and the tensor muscle of the fascia lata laterally (see also the region of the hip).

*Comment:* *At this level, the muscular body slides between the two previously mentioned muscles and forms the floor of the lateral inguinal femoral region.*

# TENSOR MUSCLE OF THE FASCIA LATA

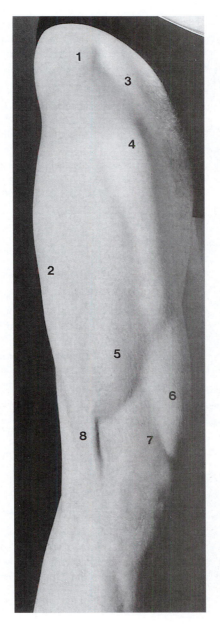

**FIGURE 4-14**
**ANTEROLATERAL VIEW OF THE THIGH**

1. Tensor muscle of the fascia lata
2. Iliotibial band
3. Sartorius muscle
4. Rectus femoris muscle
5. Vastus lateralis muscle
6. Vastus medialis muscle
7. Tendon of the quadriceps extensor muscle
8. Tendon of the iliotibial band

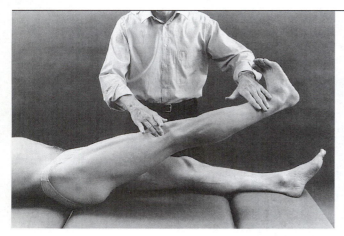

## FIGURE 4-15
### THE ILIOTIBIAL BAND IN ITS DISTAL PORTION

With the knee extended and the hip slightly flexed, create a resistance to the abduction of the hip by placing your hand over the lateral aspect of the limb just above the lateral malleolus (this technique opens up the lateral femorotibial interspace). The band is therefore under tension, since it inserts distal to the interspace mentioned previously.

In proximity to the knee, the band constitutes a strong tendon that acquires an identity of its own, particularly in male subjects.

*Comment:* *The addition of an internal rotation of the hip to the movement described above will reinforce the perception of the band in some subjects.*

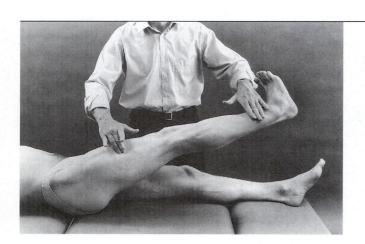

## FIGURE 4-16
### THE ILIOTIBIAL BAND AT THE LEVEL OF THE THIGH

The technical step here is the same as that described above.

It is important to remember that the band is located over the lateral aspect of the thigh and that the vastus lateralis muscle extends beyond it anteriorly and posteriorly.

*Comment:* *The resistance applied by your distal hand on the subject's leg allows a better definition of this structure.*

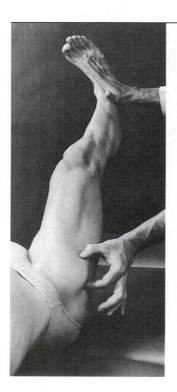

## FIGURE 4-17
### THE TENSOR MUSCLE OF THE FASCIA LATA

As shown above, with the hip in slight flexion and in internal rotation, resist, in an isometric fashion, an abduction of the hip through pressure applied against the distal aspect of the limb, just above the lateral malleolus.

In this position, the strength of the muscle is preferentially mobilized in its components of abduction and flexion of the hip; the third components (internal rotation), which the subject is asked to perform in an alternate and repetitive manner, allows a better localization of the muscular body.

In front of the gluteus medius muscle, the latter is perceived between the anterosuperior iliac spine and the anterior border of the greater trochanter.

*Comment:* *One must be careful not to confuse the tensor muscle of the fascia lata with the gluteus medius muscle. See the region of the hip. In this picture, the grip straddles the most distal portion of the muscle which is located under the gluteus medius muscle.*

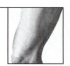

# THE POSTEROFEMORAL REGION

This region includes the medial and posterior muscular groups.

The medial muscular group consists of

- the four adductor muscles
  —the pectineus muscle (Fig. 4-20)
  —the adductor longus muscle (Fig. 4-21)
  —the adductor brevis muscle (Fig. 4-22)
  —the adductor magnus muscle (Figs. 4-23, 4-24, and 4-25)
- the gracilis muscle (Figs. 4-27, 4-28, and 4-29)

The posterior muscular group consists of

- the two medial hamstring muscles
  —the semitendinosus muscle (Figs. 4-33, 4-34, and 4-40)
  —the semimembranosus muscle (Figs. 4-35, 4-36, and 4-40)
- the lateral hamstring muscle
  —the biceps femoris muscle: the long head and the short head (Figs. 4-38, 4-39, and 4-40)

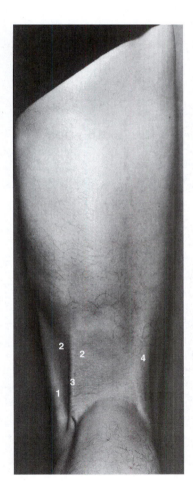

**Figure 4-18**
**Posterior view of the thigh**

1. Gracilis muscle
2. Semimembranosus muscle
3. Tendon of the semitendinosus muscle
4. Tendon of the biceps femoris muscle

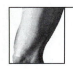
# THE MEDIAL MUSCULAR GROUP

Located in the posterofemoral region, this group includes

- the adductor muscles, composed of four muscles laid in three planes:
  —the superficial plane, formed by the pectineus muscle (Fig. 4-20) and the adductor longus muscle (Fig. 4-21)
- —the intermediate plane, formed by the adductor brevis muscle (Fig. 4-22)
  —the deep plane, formed by the adductor magnus muscle (Figs. 4-23, 4-24, and 4-25)
- the gracilis muscle (Figs. 4-27, 4-28, and 4-29)

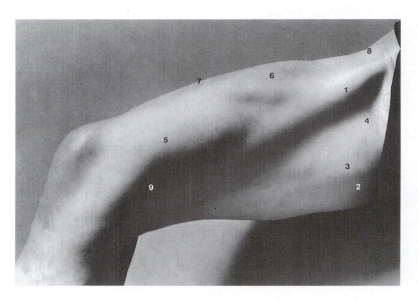

**FIGURE 4-19**
**MEDIAL VIEW OF THE THIGH**

1. Sartorius muscle
2. Gracilis muscle
3. Adductor longus muscle
4. Pectineus muscle
5. Vastus medialis muscle
6. Rectus femoris muscle
7. Vastus lateralis muscle
8. Tensor muscle of the fascia lata
9. Distal tendon of insertion of the adductor magnus muscle: insertion into the adductor tubercle on the medial condyle of the femur

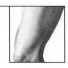

# The Adductor Muscles

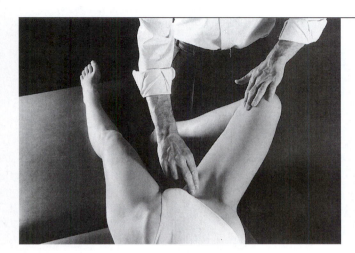

### FIGURE 4-20
### THE PECTINEUS MUSCLE

This muscle is located in front of the adductor brevis muscle, between the iliopsoas muscle laterally and the adductor longus muscle medially.

With the hip and the knee in flexion, a slight isometric resistance is opposed to an adduction of the hip. The triangular depression (with its base at the top) appearing in the proximal aspect of the thigh corresponds to the investigated muscle.

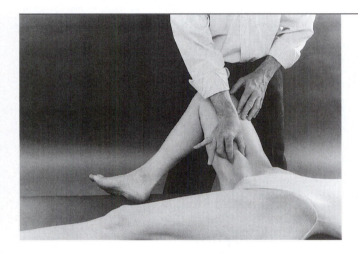

### FIGURE 4-21
### THE ADDUCTOR LONGUS MUSCLE

The hip and the knee are in flexion. The hip is also positioned in horizontal abduction. Your distal grip is placed on the medial aspect of the thigh in order to oppose resistance, through your forearm, to a horizontal adduction requested of the subject.

This double maneuver demonstrates well an important muscular mass over the medial aspect of the thigh, representing the palpated structure.

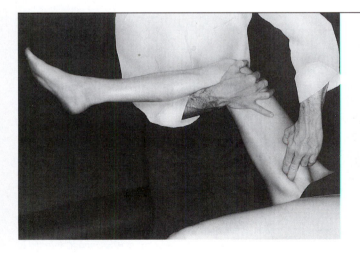

### FIGURE 4-22
### THE ADDUCTOR BREVIS MUSCLE

With one hand supporting the knee, gradually bring the hip into abduction and ask the subject to oppose a slight resistance. The gracilis muscle then appears as a cord along the medial aspect of the thigh. It is then necessary to slide your fingers between this muscle and the adductor longus muscle in the most proximal aspect of the thigh in order to come into contact with the adductor brevis muscle, particularly with its inferior bundle.

*Comment:*    *In the female subject, the adipose tissue usually covers this muscular landmark formed by the gracilis muscle. The technique of examination remains identical, simply bringing the limb in maximal abduction and then, in this extreme position, opposing a resistance to the adduction of the hip. This modification allows a better localization of the gracilis muscle in order to slide the fingers between the latter muscle and the adductor longus muscle.*

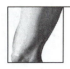

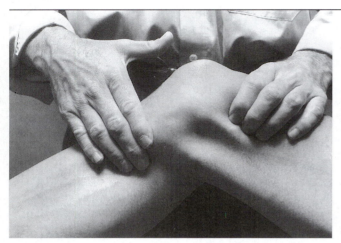

### FIGURE 4-23
### THE ADDUCTOR MAGNUS MUSCLE—MEDIAL PORTION, INFERIOR BUNDLE, OR VERTICAL BUNDLE (IN ITS DISTAL PART)

The bony landmark is the adductor tubercle (see Part III, "The Knee," which follows). The notable muscular element is the vastus medialis muscle (Fig. 4-10).

After localizing the posterior portion of the latter muscle, look for the tendon of the adductor magnus muscle, which is palpated under your fingers as a full cylindrical cord.

*Comment:* *It is possible to increase the tension of this tendon by opposing an isometric resistance to an adduction of the hip while the knee and hip are in flexion.*

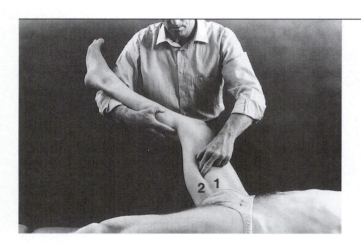

### FIGURE 4-24
### THE ADDUCTOR MAGNUS MUSCLE—LATERAL PORTION OR INTERMEDIATE BUNDLE

With one hand supporting the limb, bring the hip into abduction in order to tighten the involved adductor muscles and, more particularly, the adductor longus muscle (1) and the gracilis muscle (2). Your palpating hand slides between these two muscles as shown in this picture; it faces the lateral portion (intermediate bundle) of the adductor magnus muscle, which extends distally beyond the adductor longus muscle, and joins the middle aspect of the medial portion (or inferior bundle or vertical bundle) of the adductor magnus muscle.

### FIGURES 4-24 AND 4-25
1. Adductor longus muscle
2. Gracilis muscle

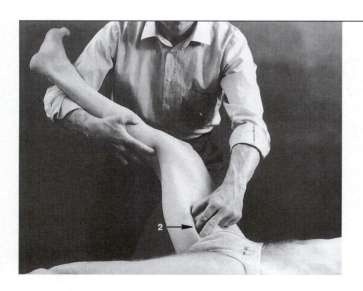

### FIGURE 4-25
### THE ADDUCTOR MAGNUS MUSCLE—MEDIAL PORTION OR VERTICAL BUNDLE AND INTERMEDIATE BUNDLE (IN ITS PROXIMAL ASPECT), POSTERIOR APPROACH

The technique of tightening the muscular landmarks is the same as that described above. With the proximal hand sliding between the adductor longus muscle (see Fig. 4-24) and the gracilis muscle (2), explore beyond the medial aspect of the thigh posteriorly in order to face the investigated structure.

*Comment:* *Remember the proximal insertion points of the involved muscular bundle, the adductor magnus muscle, into the ischial tuberosity—a very posterior structure.*

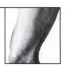

# The Gracilis Muscle

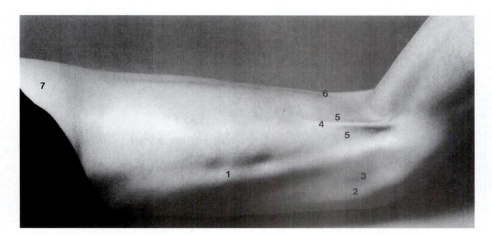

**FIGURE 4-26**
**POSTEROMEDIAL ASPECT OF THE THIGH**

1. Gracilis muscle
2. Vastus medialis muscle
3. Distal tendon of insertion of the adductor magnus muscle—insertion into the adductor tubercle on the medial condyle of the femur
4. Semitendinosus muscle
5. Semimembranosus muscle
6. Biceps femoris muscle
7. Gluteus maximus muscle

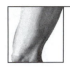
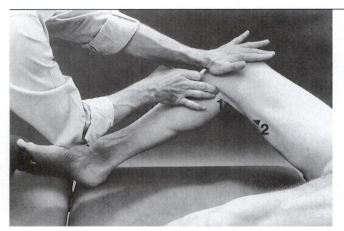

### FIGURE 4-27
### THE GRACILIS MUSCLE IN ITS DISTAL PORTION OVER THE MEDIAL BORDER OF THE TIBIA

The subject is supine with the hip and knee in flexion. Ask the subject to perform a medial rotation as well as an isometric flexion of the knee (by pushing the heel against the table and toward the buttock). Your grip is placed over the medial border of the tibia, your middle finger is placed against the investigated tendon, and your ring finger faces the semitendinosus muscle (1). The semimembranosus muscle (2) appears in the distal half of the thigh between these two tendons.

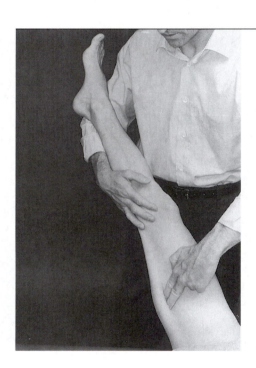

### FIGURE 4-28
### THE GRACILIS MUSCLE AT THE THIGH LEVEL

Your distal hand supports the limb and brings the hip into abduction. Ask the subject to perform an adduction of the hip while resisting this movement in order to protrude the muscular body, which is more or less visible depending on the individual subject.

As shown in this figure, this muscle may be lifted off the underlying muscular planes with a bidigital grip.

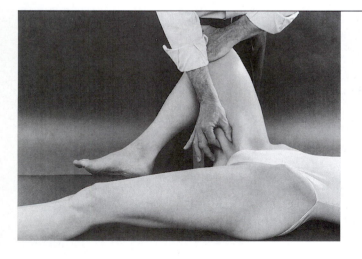

### FIGURE 4-29
### THE GRACILIS MUSCLE IN ITS PROXIMAL ASPECT

The subject's knee is in flexion while the hip is positioned in flexion and in external rotation. Your distal hand is positioned against the medial aspect of the knee in order to resist a horizontal adduction of the hip. Your proximal hand grabs the examined muscle over the medial aspect of the thigh.

*Comment:*   *In the female subject, the amount of adipose tissue in this region may hamper the examination.*

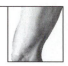

# THE POSTERIOR MUSCULAR GROUP

Located in the posterofemoral region, this group includes

- the medial hamstring muscles, composed of two muscles:
  —the semitendinosus muscle (Figs. 4-33, 4-34, and 4-40)
  —the semimembranosus muscle (Figs. 4-35, 4-36, and 4-40)

- the lateral hamstring muscle, composed of
  —the biceps femoris muscle:
    • long head
    • short head (Figs. 4-38, 4-39, and 4-40)

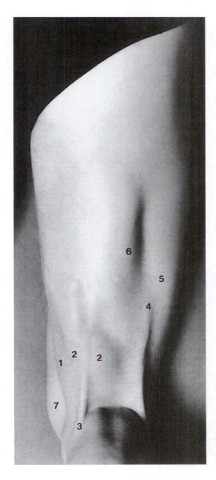

**FIGURE 4-30**
**POSTERIOR VIEW OF THE THIGH**

1. Gracilis muscle
2. Semimembranosus muscle
3. Semitendinosus muscle
4. Tendon of the biceps femoris muscle
5. Short head of the biceps
6. Long head of the biceps
7. Vastus medialis muscle

# THE MEDIAL HAMSTRING MUSCLES

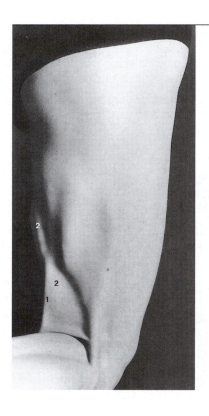

**FIGURE 4-31**
**POSTEROLATERAL VIEW OF THE THIGH**

1. Semitendinosus muscle

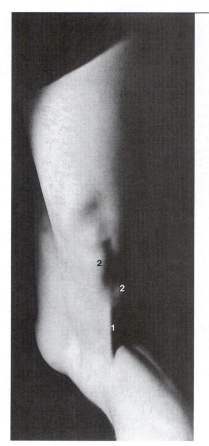

**FIGURE 4-32**
**POSTEROMEDIAL VIEW OF THE THIGH**

2. Semimembranosus muscle

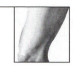

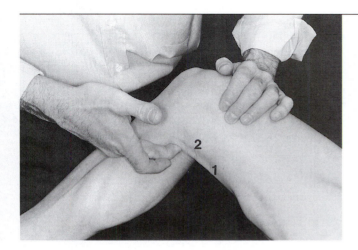

### Figure 4-33
### THE TENDON OF THE SEMITENDINOSUS MUSCLE OVER THE MEDIAL BORDER OF THE TIBIA

In this figure, a digital grip is placed against the medial border of the tibia and your middle finger hooks up the tendon of the semitendinosus muscle (1). In this position (knee in flexion), the tendon of the gracilis muscle (2) is located in front of the tendon of the semitendinosus muscle.

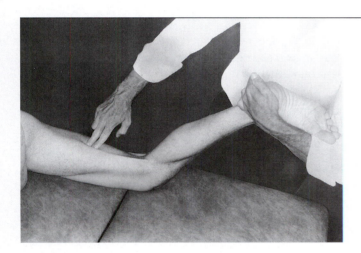

### Figure 4-34
### THE SEMITENDINOSUS MUSCLE OVER THE POSTERIOR ASPECT OF THE THIGH

Your distal hand covers the heel and leans over the medial aspect of the foot in order to resist a simultaneous flexion and internal rotation of the knee. The body of the muscle is found in the extension of its tendon (Fig. 4-33).

The muscle is located in the posterior part of the thigh, medial to the biceps femoris muscle and behind the semimembranosus muscle.

*Comment:*   *A particular aspect of this muscle is that its tendon extends proximally over the posterior aspect of the thigh, as clearly shown in this figure.*

*With regard to its proximal insertion into the ischial tuberosity, see Fig. 4-40.*

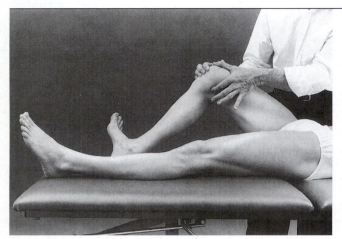

**FIGURE 4-35**

**THE SEMIMEMBRANOSUS MUSCLE IN ITS DISTAL ASPECT: MEDIAL VIEW**

Your distal hand brings the leg into external rotation in order to isolate the distal end of the tendon. The latter is palpated as a large, cylindrical cord near its insertion into the postero-medial aspect of the proximal end of the medial condyle of the tibia.

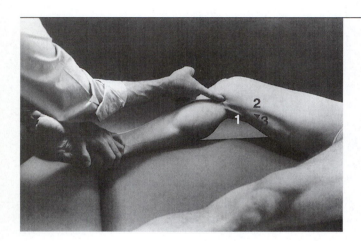

**FIGURE 4-36**

**THE SEMIMEMBRANOSUS MUSCLE IN ITS DISTAL ASPECT: POSTEROMEDIAL VIEW**

In addition to the technique described above, you may ask the subject to perform a flexion and internal rotation of the knee while he or she opposes some resistance in order to better perceive the tendon under the finger.

*Comment:* *With your index finger placed against the semimembranosus muscle at its insertion into the tibia, note that the gracilis muscle (2) runs across it posteriorly to position itself above the semitendinosus muscle (1), over the medial border of the tibia.*

# The Lateral Hamstring Muscle

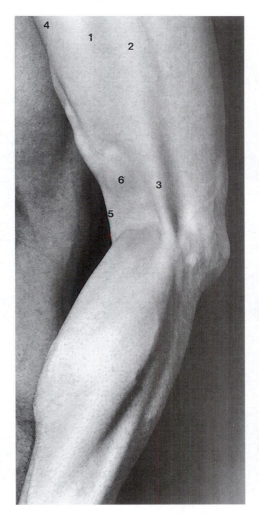

**FIGURE 4-37**
**POSTEROLATERAL VIEW OF THE THIGH**

1. Biceps femoris muscle—long head
2. Biceps femoris muscle—short head
3. Tendon of the biceps femoris muscle
4. Semitendinosus muscle
5. Tendon of the semitendinosus muscle
6. Semimembranosus muscle

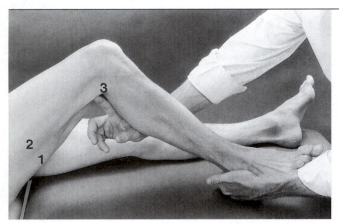

### FIGURE 4-38

### THE BICEPS FEMORIS MUSCLE IN ITS DISTAL ASPECT

Your hand, covering the heel, resists a flexion of the knee, while you apply the anterior aspect of your forearm against the lateral border of the foot, resisting an external rotation of the knee.

The tendon is demonstrated over the lateral aspect of the knee, just proximal to its insertion into the head of the fibula.

*Comment:*   *The fibers of the long head of the biceps femoris muscle (1) end in the anterior portion of the tendon (3), while the fibers of the short head (2) also end in the anterior surface of this tendon (3), but over its lateral border.*

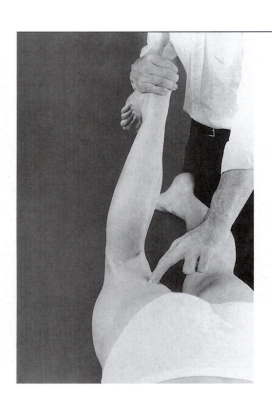

### FIGURE 4-39

### THE BICEPS FEMORIS MUSCLE OVER THE POSTERIOR ASPECT OF THE THIGH

With the subject in prone position, your distal hand covers the heel and is placed against the lateral border of the foot in order to resist the flexion and external rotation of the knee. Over the posterior aspect of the thigh, the long and short heads of the biceps femoris muscle join the medial hamstring muscles.

---

### FIGURES 4-38 AND 4-40

1. Biceps femoris muscle—long head
2. Biceps femoris muscle—short head
3. Tendon of the biceps femoris muscle
4. Gluteal fold

---

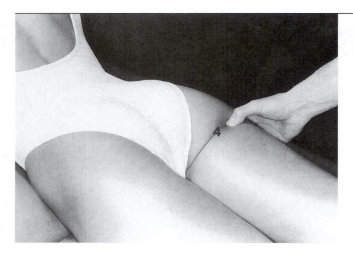

### FIGURE 4-40

### TENDONS OF THE HAMSTRING MUSCLES INSERTING INTO THE ISCHIAL TUBEROSITY

The subject is in prone position and the essential landmark is the gluteal fold (4).

You can palpate muscular insertions into the ischial tuberosity through this fold.

For more details, refer to the pages dedicated to the involved muscles: the semitendinosus muscle (page 53), the semimembranosus muscle (page 54), and the biceps femoris muscle (this page). It might be interesting to offer resistance to the flexion of the knee for a better perception by the thumb of the tightening of these tendons.

# THE
# KNEE

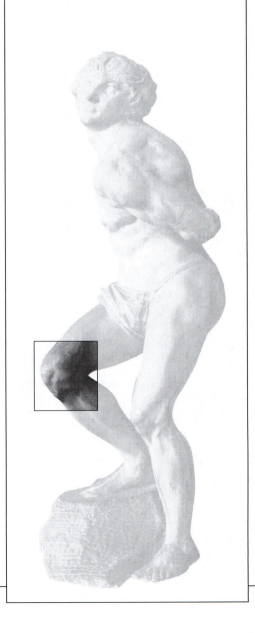

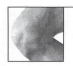

# ILLUSTRATED STUDY OF THE KNEE (ANTERIOR)

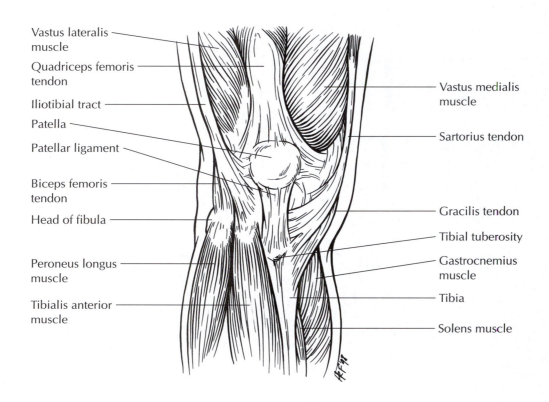

Vastus lateralis muscle

Quadriceps femoris tendon

Iliotibial tract

Patella

Patellar ligament

Biceps femoris tendon

Head of fibula

Peroneus longus muscle

Tibialis anterior muscle

Vastus medialis muscle

Sartorius tendon

Gracilis tendon

Tibial tuberosity

Gastrocnemius muscle

Tibia

Solens muscle

# ILLUSTRATED STUDY OF THE KNEE (POSTERIOR)

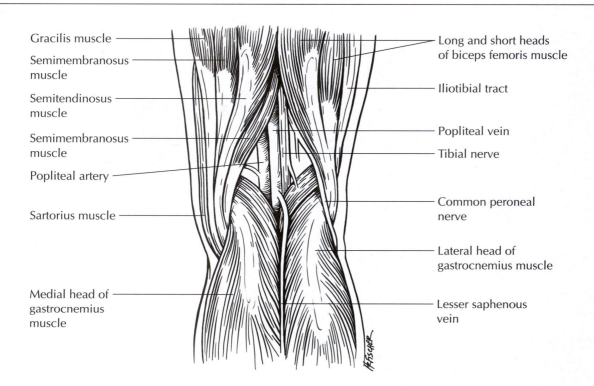

Gracilis muscle

Semimembranosus muscle

Semitendinosus muscle

Semimembranosus muscle

Popliteal artery

Sartorius muscle

Medial head of gastrocnemius muscle

Long and short heads of biceps femoris muscle

Iliotibial tract

Popliteal vein

Tibial nerve

Common peroneal nerve

Lateral head of gastrocnemius muscle

Lesser saphenous vein

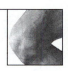

# ILLUSTRATED STUDY OF THE KNEE (LATERAL)

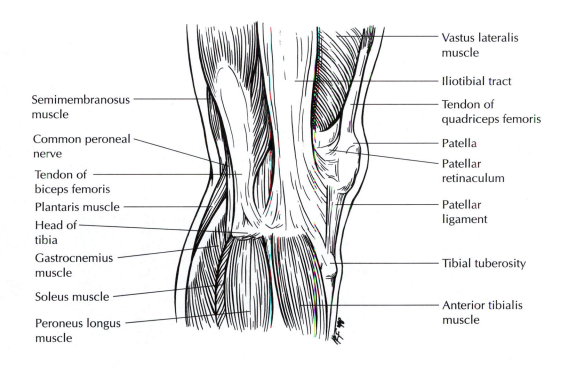

Semimembranosus muscle

Common peroneal nerve

Tendon of biceps femoris

Plantaris muscle

Head of tibia

Gastrocnemius muscle

Soleus muscle

Peroneus longus muscle

Vastus lateralis muscle

Iliotibial tract

Tendon of quadriceps femoris

Patella

Patellar retinaculum

Patellar ligament

Tibial tuberosity

Anterior tibialis muscle

# ILLUSTRATED STUDY OF THE KNEE (MEDIAL)

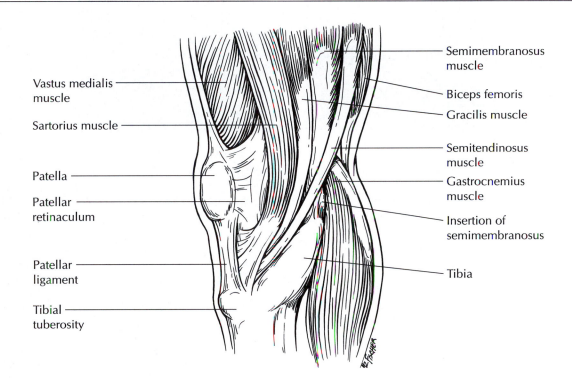

Vastus medialis muscle

Sartorius muscle

Patella

Patellar retinaculum

Patellar ligament

Tibial tuberosity

Semimembranosus muscle

Biceps femoris

Gracilis muscle

Semitendinosus muscle

Gastrocnemius muscle

Insertion of semimembranosus

Tibia

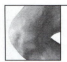
## TOPOGRAPHIC PRESENTATION OF THE KNEE

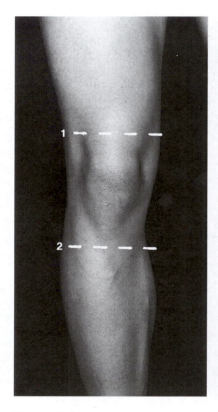

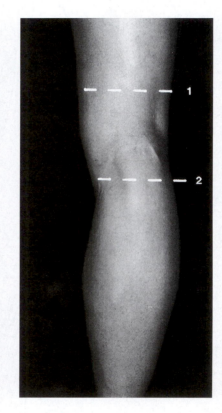

**FIGURE 5-1**
**ANTERIOR VIEW**

1.  Superior border

**FIGURE 5-2**
**POSTERIOR VIEW**

2.  Inferior border

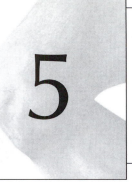

# 5

# OSTEOLOGY

## THE ANTERIOR COMPARTMENT

The bony structures accessible by palpation are as follows:

- the suprapatellar fossa (Fig. 5-4)
- the patella
  —the base of the patella (Fig. 5-5)
  —the anterior surface (Fig. 5-6)
  —the apex (Fig. 5-7)
  —the lateral borders (Fig. 5-8)
  —the lateral approach to the posterior surface (Fig. 5-9)
  —the medial approach to the posterior surface (Fig. 5-10)

- the femur
  —the articular surfaces of the medial and lateral condyles (Fig. 5-13)
  —the trochleocondylar grooves (Figs. 5-14 and 5-15)
- the tibia
  —the tibial plateau and the femorotibial articular interspace (Fig. 5-12)
  —the anterior tuberosity of the tibia (Fig. 5-11)

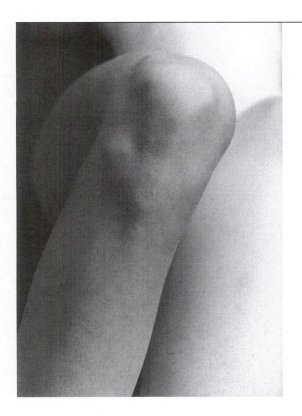

**FIGURE 5-3**
**FRONTAL VIEW — KNEE IN FLEXION**

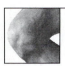

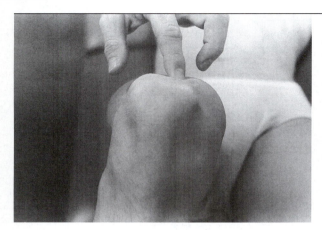

## FIGURE 5-4
### THE SUPRAPATELLAR FOSSA OF THE FEMUR

Located above the condyles, at the level of the anterior aspect of the lower extremity of the femur, this area is triangular in shape and accepts the upper part of the patella during extension.

The knee must be maximally flexed in order to facilitate its palpation, starting at the base of the patella, which is easily found (see Fig. 5-5, below).

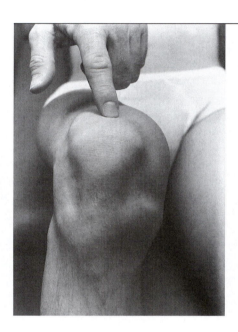

## FIGURE 5-5
### THE BASE OF THE PATELLA

This triangular area, with a large anterior base and a posterior apex, is palpated as a sloped surface.

*Comment:*     *The base of the patella is a site of insertion of the tendon of the quadriceps extensor muscle anteriorly and of the articular capsule posteriorly, near its articular surface.*

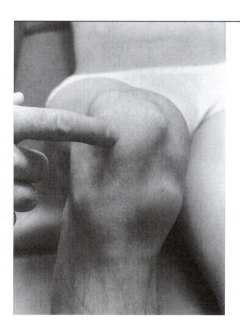

## FIGURE 5-6
### THE ANTERIOR SURFACE OF THE PATELLA

Convex and perforated by numerous vascular apertures, this surface is rough; it consists of vertical striae formed by the tendon of the quadriceps extensor muscle.

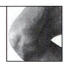

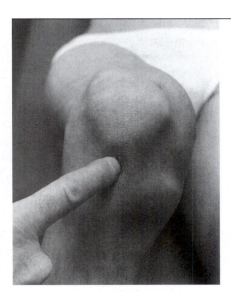

## Figure 5-7
### The apex of the patella

This area is pointed toward the distal aspect of the limb; the patellar ligament is attached to it. It is possible to approach it with the knee in flexion or in extension.

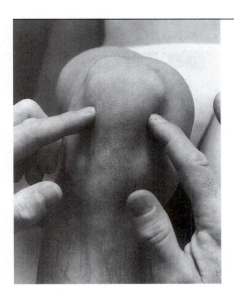

## Figure 5-8
### The lateral borders of the patella

The medial and lateral borders are directed from above downward and medially if one refers to the median axis of the patella. They are directly accessible by palpation.

*Comment:*   *It is at the level of the junction of these borders with the base of the patella that the attachment of the corresponding patellar retinaculum is found.*

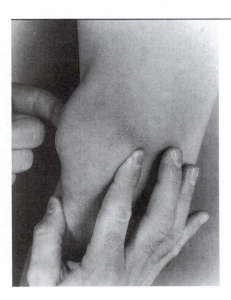

## Figure 5-9
### Lateral approach to the posterior surface of the patella

Only the lateralmost aspect of this facet is accessible. With the knee in hyperextension and the quadriceps extensor muscle completely relaxed, the patella should be pushed laterally.

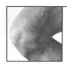

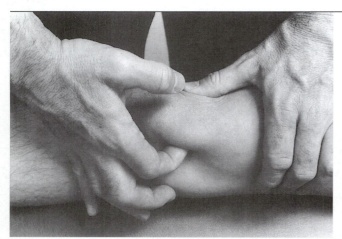

### FIGURE 5-10
### MEDIAL APPROACH TO THE POSTERIOR SURFACE
### OF THE PATELLA

With the knee in hyperextension and the quadriceps extensor muscle completely relaxed, the patella should be pushed medially.

*Comment:*     *Less concave than the lateral facet, the medial facet is in contact with the medial condyle of the femur. It is, in fact, composed of two articular surfaces.*

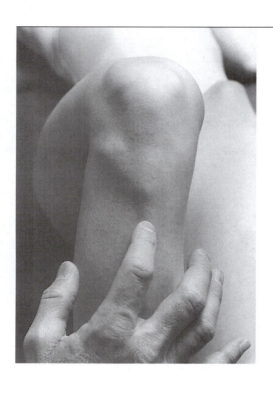

### FIGURE 5-11
### THE ANTERIOR TUBEROSITY OF THE TIBIA

This triangular surface, with a distal apex, separates the medial and lateral condyles of the tibia anteriorly.

It is easy to delineate and is the site of insertion of the patellar ligament.

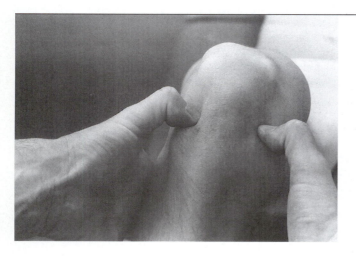

### FIGURE 5-12
### THE TIBIAL PLATEAU

With the knee flexed at 90°, your thumbs should be positioned on each side of the patellar ligament and the femorotibial articular interspace. The thumbs should be brought downward in order to be in contact with the nonarticular anterior border of this plateau (palpate its border up to its junction with the femur).

*Comment:*     *This grip also permits examination of the femorotibial articular interspace.*

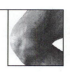

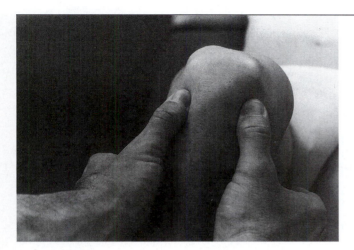

### FIGURE 5-13

### THE ARTICULAR SURFACES OF THE MEDIAL AND LATERAL CONDYLES OF THE FEMUR

With the knee flexed at 90°, your thumbs should be positioned on each side of the patellar ligament in the femorotibial articular interspace. The thumbs should be lifted upward in order to contact the investigated structures. If any difficulty is encountered, an increased degree of flexion of the knee will facilitate this examination.

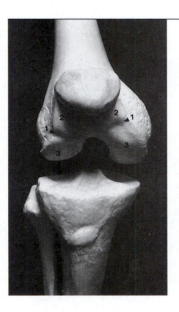

### FIGURE 5-14

### VISUALIZATION OF THE TROCHLEOCONDYLAR GROOVES OF THE FEMUR

These grooves are shaped by the articular surface of the inferior extremity of the femur, which is covered by cartilage in two parts. The articular surfaces located anteriorly above these grooves are part of the trochlea. The articular surfaces located posteriorly and under these grooves are called the articular surfaces of the condyles.

1.   Trochleocondylar grooves
2.   Trochlea of the femur
3.   Articular surfaces of the medial and lateral condyles

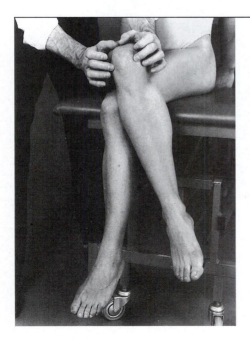

### FIGURE 5-15

### APPROACH TO THE TROCHLEOCONDYLAR GROOVES

The ideal position is a knee flexed at slightly more than 90°. Using a digital grip, follow the articular surface between the patella and the articular surfaces of the condyles in order to perceive these two grooves or depressions, called the trochleocondylar grooves (see Fig. 5-14) (1).

*Comment:*    *The medial trochleocondylar groove is often palpated much more easily.*

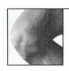

# THE MEDIAL COMPARTMENT

The bony structures accessible by palpation are as follows:

- the femur
  —the tuberosity of the medial condyle (Figs. 5-17 and 5-18)
  —the medial border of the medial aspect of the articular surface of the medial condyle (Fig. 5-19)
  —the medial supracondylar groove (Fig. 5-19)
  —the medial trochleocondylar articular surface (Fig. 5-20)
  —the adductor tubercle (Fig. 5-21)

- the tibia
  —the medial tibial plateau (Fig. 5-22)
  —the inferior border of the medial condyle of the tibia (Fig. 5-23)
  —the superior portion of the medial border of the tibia [structure notable for the localization of the pes anserinus muscles (Fig. 5-24)]

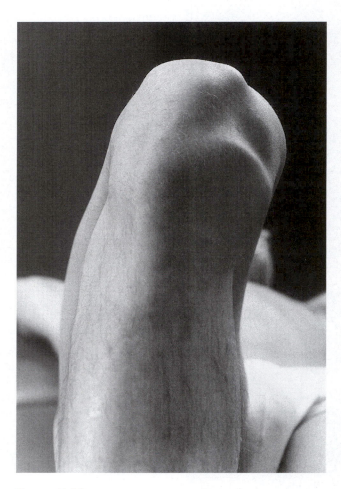

**FIGURE 5-16**
**ANTEROMEDIAL VIEW—KNEE IN FLEXION**

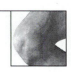

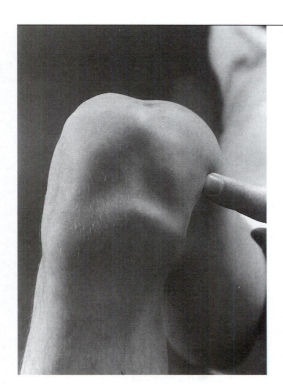

## FIGURE 5-17
### THE MEDIAL EPICONDYLE OF THE FEMUR—ANTERIOR VIEW

This subcutaneous structure, which is directly accessible by palpation, is the most prominent bony structure of the rough medial surface of the medial condyle.

*Comment:*     *On its posterior aspect is a depression for the insertion of the tibial collateral ligament of the knee.*

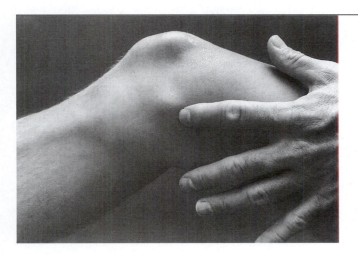

## FIGURE 5-18
### THE MEDIAL EPICONDYLE OF THE FEMUR—MEDIAL VIEW

This medial view of the medial epicondyle allows better visualization and localization of the investigated structure.

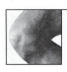

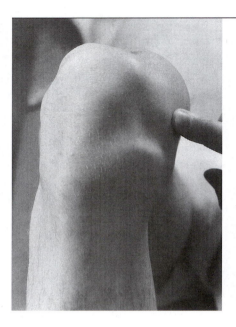

## FIGURE 5-19
### THE MEDIAL BORDER OF THE MEDIAL ASPECT OF THE MEDIAL TROCHLEOCONDYLAR ARTICULAR SURFACE OF THE FEMUR

This border is the medial boundary for the femoral condyle and the articular surface of the medial condyle. A maximal flexion of the knee facilitates its access.

### The medial supracondylar groove

Inferiorly, this structure lines the rough lateral surface of the medial condyle of the femur. Its depth is more pronounced in the back than in the front.

Position the knee in flexion to free it from the musculotendinous structures.

*Comment:*     *Do not forget that when the knee is flexed, a large portion of the inferior articular surface of the femur is exposed.*

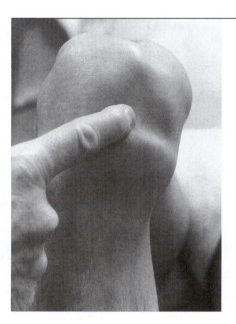

## FIGURE 5-20
### THE MEDIAL TROCHLEOCONDYLAR ARTICULAR SURFACE OF THE FEMUR

With your thumb and index finger, locate the medial femorotibial articular interspace.

From this landmark, follow the articular surface, which is palpated as a smooth surface under your finger. This articular surface is limited by the medial border of the medial trochleocondylar articular surface.

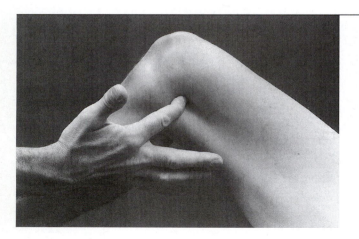

## FIGURE 5-21
### THE ADDUCTOR TUBERCLE

Although the investigation of this structure is in itself somewhat difficult, it is possible to locate it by first finding the vertical tendon of the adductor magnus muscle (see Fig. 7-18) and following this tendon to its distal end, where a bony prominence represents the investigated structure.

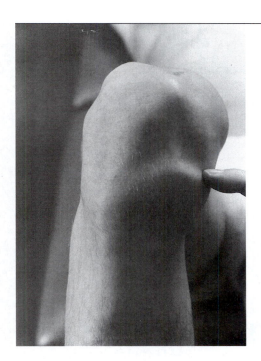

## Figure 5-22
### The medial tibial plateau

With the knee flexed at 90°, this area is easy to locate. From an anterior view, the medial aspect of the plateau is interesting to visualize, since the tibial collateral ligament is approached from it.

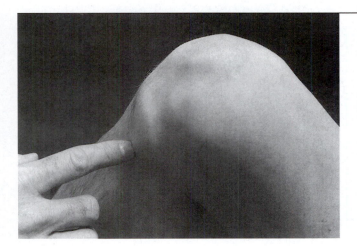

## Figure 5-23
### The inferior border of the medial condyle of the tibia

With the knee in flexion, the medial border of the tibia should be located and followed to its upper extremity. The medial tuberosity can then be easily palpated by a hook type of digital grip.

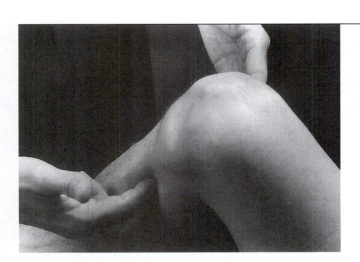

## Figure 5-24
### The proximal aspect of the medial border of the tibia

This bony structure is noteworthy because it is where the pes anserinus muscles (the semitendinosus, gracilis, and sartorius muscles) are located.

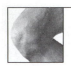

# THE EXTERNAL COMPARTMENT

The accessible bony structures by palpation are as follows:

- the femur
  —the lateral border of the suprapatellar fossa (Fig. 5-26)
  —the lateral border of the lateral aspect of the lateral trochleocondylar articular surface (Fig. 5-27)
  —the lateral epicondyle of the femur (Fig. 5-28)
  —the lateral supracondylar groove (Fig. 5-29)
  —the lateral trochleocondylar articular surface (Figs. 5-29 and 5-30)

- the tibia
  —the lateral tibial plateau (Fig. 5-31)
  —the lateral condyle (Figs. 5-32 and 5-33)
  —the oblique crest (Fig. 5-34)
- the fibula
  —the head (Fig. 5-35)
  —the neck (Fig. 5-36)

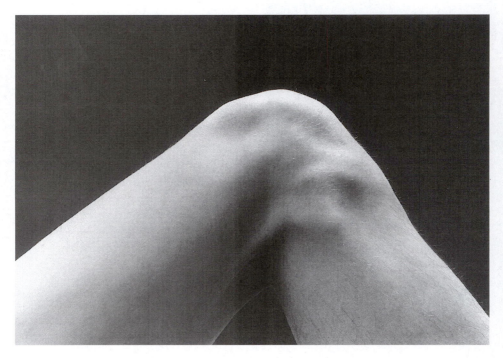

**FIGURE 5-25**
**LATERAL VIEW—KNEE IN FLEXION**

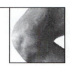

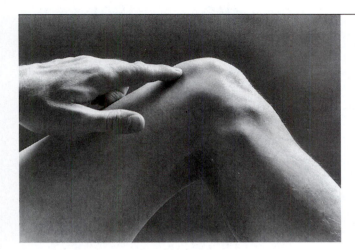

### FIGURE 5-26
### THE LATERAL BORDER OF THE SUPRAPATELLAR FOSSA

This is more pronounced than the medial border and becomes even more obvious as the knee is gradually brought into maximal flexion.

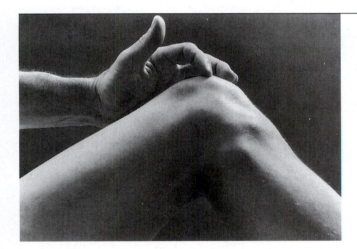

### FIGURE 5-27
### THE LATERAL BORDER OF THE LATERAL ASPECT OF THE LATERAL TROCHLEOCONDYLAR ARTICULAR SURFACE OF THE FEMUR

Its very lateral position reveals the off-center positioning of the patella when the knee is flexed.

*Comment:*     *Consequently, the trochleocondylar surface is more exposed on its medial than on its lateral aspect when the knee is flexed.*

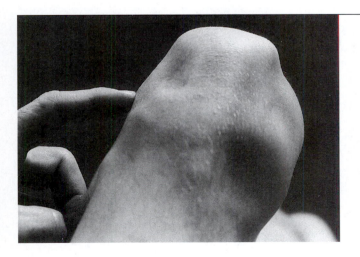

### FIGURE 5-28
### THE LATERAL EPICONDYLE OF THE FEMUR

Much less prominent than the medial tuberosity, this epicondyle is located over the middle aspect of the lateral surface of the condyle.

In case of difficulty in locating it, place the fibular collateral ligament under tension by opening the lateral femorotibial articular interspace with the subject's knee in flexion (see Fig. 3-39). The tuberosity is located above the point of insertion of the ligament mentioned above into the femur.

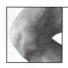

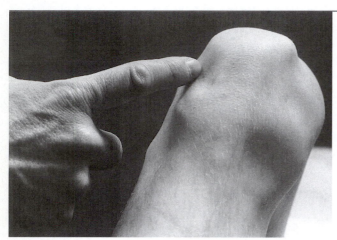

## FIGURE 5-29

### THE LATERAL BORDER OF THE LATERAL ASPECT OF THE LATERAL TROCHLEOCONDYLAR ARTICULAR SURFACE OF THE FEMUR

This border delineates the femoral trochlea laterally and the articular surface of the lateral condyle. A maximal flexion of the knee facilitates its access.

### THE LATERAL SUPRACONDYLAR GROOVE

This area is lined inferiorly by the rough lateral surface of the lateral condyle. The depth of the groove is more pronounced in the back than in the front.

Position the knee in flexion in order to free it from the musculotendinous structures.

*Comment:* **Do not forget that when the knee is flexed, the inferior extremity of the femur is exposed.**

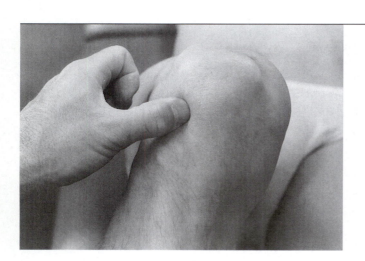

## FIGURE 5-30

### THE LATERAL ASPECT OF THE LATERAL TROCHLEOCONDYLAR ARTICULAR SURFACE OF THE FEMUR

Using your thumb, locate the lateral femorotibial articular interspace. From this landmark, follow the articular surface, which is felt as a smooth surface. This articular surface is limited medially by the patellar ligament and the lateral border of the patella. It is limited laterally by the lateral border of the lateral trochleocondylar articular surface.

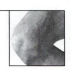

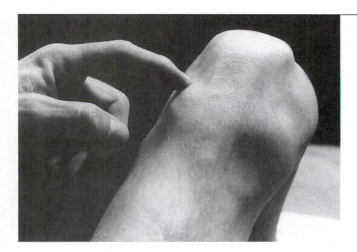

### FIGURE 5-31
### THE LATERAL TIBIAL PLATEAU

With the knee in flexion at 90°, this plateau is located without difficulty. In an anterior view, it is interesting to visualize the most lateral portion of the plateau, where the fibular collateral ligament is approached at the level of the articular interspace.

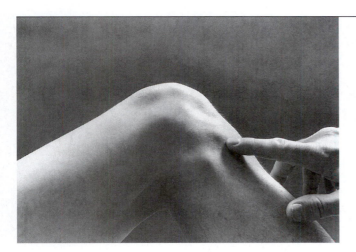

### FIGURE 5-32
### THE TUBERCLE OF THE LATERAL CONDYLE OF THE TIBIA (GERDY) — LATERAL VIEW

This is the most prominent structure of the lateral tuberosity of the tibia. With the knee in flexion at 90°, it is examined just under the lateral aspect of the tibial plateau and lateral to the tibial tuberosity.

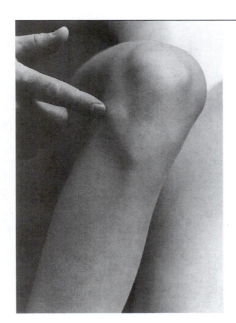

### FIGURE 5-33
### THE TUBERCLE OF THE LATERAL CONDYLE OF THE TIBIA (GERDY) — ANTERIOR VIEW

A complementary anterior view allows a more precise visualization and localization of this structure. An additional bony landmark is offered by the head of the fibula, which is located behind and distal to the investigated structure.

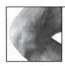

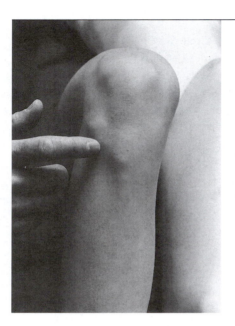

**FIGURE 5-34**
**"THE OBLIQUE CREST" OF THE TIBIA—FRONTAL VIEW**

This is a bony crest extending from the tubercle of the lateral tuberosity of the tibia (Gerdy) (see Figs. 5-32 and 5-33) and the lateral border of the tibial tuberosity (see Fig. 5-13). It is oblique and directed downward and forward. It is directly accessible under the skin.

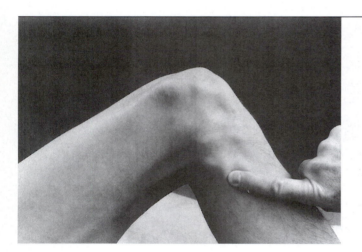

**FIGURE 5-35**
**THE HEAD OF THE FIBULA—LATERAL VIEW**

Access to the head of the fibula is very easy. To make it more prominent, the leg may be rotated internally.

*Comment:*    *The styloid process is a bony prominence that projects behind and lateral to the articular surface of the head of the fibula.*

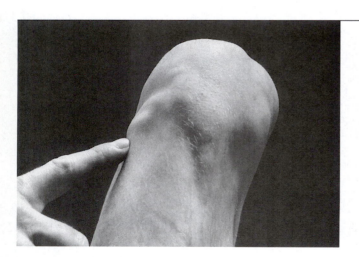

**FIGURE 5-36**
**THE NECK OF THE FIBULA—FRONTAL VIEW**

This structure, which is interposed between the head and the shaft of the fibula, is noteworthy, since the common peroneal nerve passes around it before entering the leg.

# 6

# ARTHROLOGY: THE ARTICULATIONS

## THE LIGAMENTS

The ligaments that are accessible by palpation are as follows:

- the fibular collateral ligament: visualization and placement under tension (Figs. 6-2 and 6-3)
- "the lateral patellar retinaculum": placement under tension (Figs. 6-4, 6-5, and 6-6)
- the tibial collateral ligament: visualization and placement under tension (Figs. 6-7 through 6-10)

- "the medial patellar retinaculum": (Figs. 6-11, 6-12, and 6-13)
- the infrapatellar adipose tissue: visualization and approach (Fig. 6-14)
- the patellar ligament (Fig. 6-15)

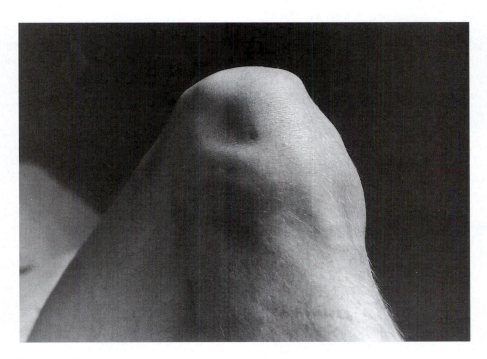

**FIGURE 6-1**
**ANTERIOR VIEW OF THE KNEE**

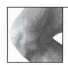

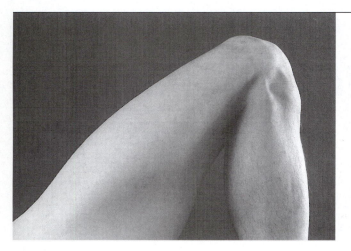

### FIGURE 6-2
### VISUALIZATION OF THE FIBULAR COLLATERAL LIGAMENT

This ligament extends from the lateral tuberosity of the femur down the anterolateral aspect of the head of the fibula, in front of the styloid process.

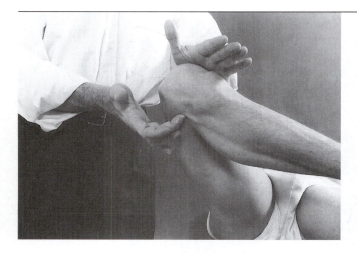

### FIGURE 6-3
### PLACEMENT UNDER TENSION OF THE FIBULAR COLLATERAL LIGAMENT

For optimal localization, place the fibular collateral ligament under tension. Once it is located, its examination is facilitated in any position of the knee.

Position the subject as shown in this figure. Apply some pressure from inside out, using one hand positioned over the medial aspect of the knee in order to open up the lateral articular interspace, which places the ligament under tension. The other hand faces the lateral articular interspace, between the head of the fibula and the lateral tuberosity of the femur.

*Comment:* ***The ligament is palpated as a full cylindrical cord. Its thickness varies from person to person. Individuals with a varus deformity of the knee will obviously have a much stronger and thicker ligament, since it is constantly mobilized.***

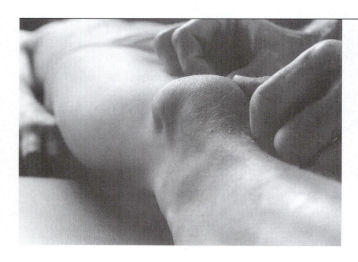

### FIGURE 6-4
### VISUALIZATION OF THE LATERAL PATELLAR RETINACULUM, TRANSVERSE BUNDLE

The knee is in complete extension and the extensor quadriceps muscle is relaxed. The patella may either be pushed laterally, which places the investigated structure under tension (see figure), or be pushed medially, which has the same effect. The lateral patellar retinaculum is approached in a plane perpendicular to its course.

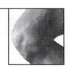

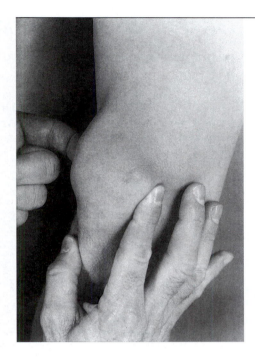

## FIGURE 6-5
### PALPATION OF THE LATERAL PATELLAR RETINACULUM, TRANSVERSE BUNDLE

This maneuver brings the structure investigated and visualized in Fig. 6-4 into a plane that is closer to the strict sagittal plane. It is a capsular reinforcement that is palpated as a fibrous band.

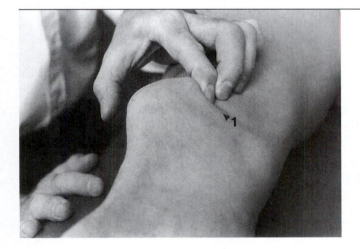

## FIGURE 6-6
### VISUALIZATION OF THE PLACEMENT UNDER TENSION OF BOTH THE MEDIAL AND THE LATERAL PATELLAR RETINACULAE

An outward traction of the patella allows the examiner to create a projection of the medial patellar retinaculum (1) and, at the same time, to put under tension the lateral patellar retinaculum, not visible in this figure (see Fig. 6-4).

*Comment:* *During this maneuver, the lateral patellar retinaculum is brought under tension in a plane that moves progressively closer to the strict sagittal plane, while the medial patellar retinaculum is brought under tension in a more and more horizontal plane. This figure presents an inferomedial view.*

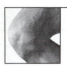
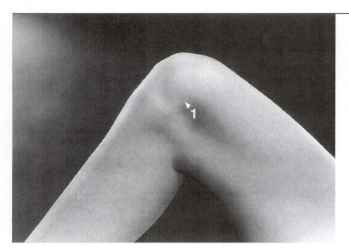

**FIGURE 6-7**

**VISUALIZATION OF THE TIBIAL COLLATERAL LIGAMENT**

This ligament (1) extends from the superior aspect of the medial tuberosity of the femur. It is also inserted into a depression located just behind this tuberosity down to the superior portion of the internal border of the tibia and to the adjacent portion of the anteromedial surface of the same bone.

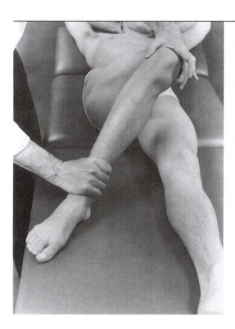

**FIGURE 6-8**

**PLACEMENT UNDER TENSION OF THE TIBIAL COLLATERAL LIGAMENT**

The optimal placement of this ligament under tension is carried out in two steps. With the subject's knee flexed at 90°, the leg is first brought into external rotation, which puts the ligament under tension.

As a second step, push the knee medially (while the foot is immobilized on the table) with one hand. This opens up the medial articular interspace and increases the tension on the investigated structure.

*Comment:* **The fingers of the same hand facing the articular interspace perceive the ligament as a relatively flat fibrous band.**

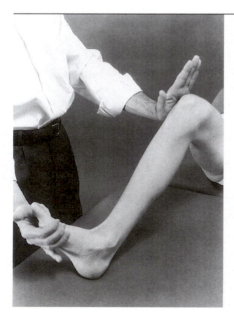

**FIGURE 6-9**

**ALTERNATIVE TECHNIQUE TO PLACE THE TIBIAL COLLATERAL LIGAMENT UNDER TENSION**

With the heel leaning on the table, grab the medial aspect of the foot in order to bring the leg into external rotation.

As a second step, the other hand applies pressure against the lateral aspect of the knee and moves the knee medially, opening up the medial articular interspace and therefore putting the ligament under tension.

*Comment:* **The ligament is clearly demonstrated at the level of the medial articular interspace (see Fig. 6-10).**

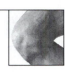

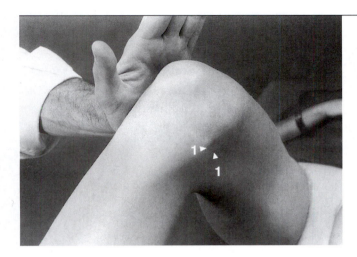

## Figure 6-10

### As an alternative technique to place the tibial collateral ligament under tension, maneuver as in the previous figure, closeup view

This picture demonstrates an anteromedial closeup view of the knee, clearly showing the placement of the tibial collateral ligament under tension.

*Comment:*   ***The ligament is clearly demonstrated at the level of the medial articular interspace (1).***

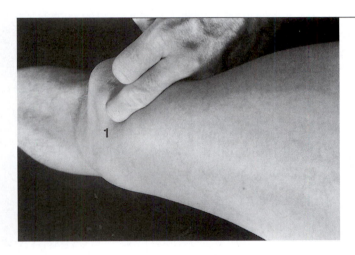

## Figure 6-11

### Visualization of the medial patellar retinaculum, transverse bundle — medial view with knee in extension

With the knee in complete extension, the quadriceps extensor muscle is relaxed. The patella may be either pushed laterally, which puts the ligament under tension (see figure), or pushed medially (Fig. 6-12), which also puts the ligament under tension.

Palpation is the same in both cases. The medial patellar retinaculum is approached transversely.

1.   Medial patellar retinaculum

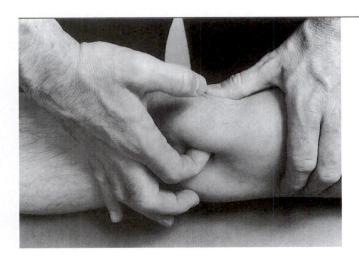

## Figure 6-12

### Palpation of the medial patellar retinaculum, transverse bundle

This maneuver puts the investigated structure under tension in a plane that is closer to the sagittal plane. It is a capsular reinforcement, which is palpated as a fibrous band.

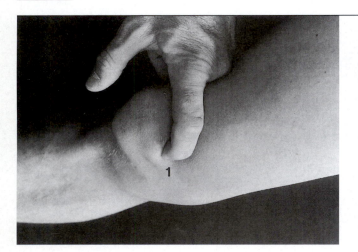

## FIGURE 6-13
### PLACEMENT UNDER TENSION OF THE MEDIAL PATELLAR RETINACULUM, TRANSVERSE BUNDLE, BY OUTWARD TRACTION OF THE PATELLA

This maneuver, the same as that described in Fig. 6-6, tightens up the examined structure in a plane that is closer and closer to the horizontal plane. This is a capsular reinforcement which is palpated as a fibrous band.

1. Medial patellar retinaculum

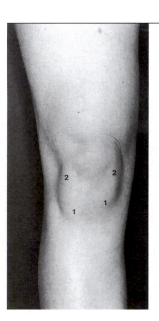

## FIGURE 6-14
### VISUALIZATION OF THE INFRAPATELLAR ADIPOSE TISSUE

Located between the patellar ligament and the nonarticular posterior aspect of the patella, this structure is found above the intercondylar aspect of the tibial plateau. This adipose tissue extends medially and laterally to the middle aspect of the lateral borders of the patella, forming rolls of fat also called *plicae alares*. They are seen more easily during extension of the knee, as shown in the figure.

1. Infrapatellar adipose tissue
2. Infrapatellar adipose tissue: plicae alares

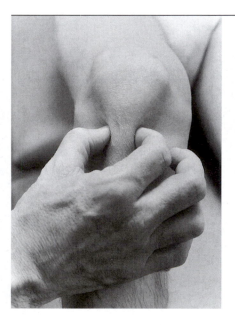

## FIGURE 6-15
### THE PATELLAR LIGAMENT

This ligament may be approached with the knee either flexed or in extension. Grab the medial and lateral borders of this ligament by a thumb–index finger grip. The ligament's slightly oblique downward and forward course is then better perceived.

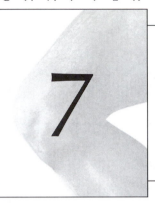

# 7

# MYOLOGY

## THE ANTEROLATERAL REGION

The muscular and tendinous structures accessible by palpation are as follows below.

Involving the thigh:
- the vastus lateralis muscle (Fig. 7-2)
- the iliotibial tract or Maissiat's band (Fig. 7-3)
- the tendon of the biceps femoris muscle (Fig. 7-4)

Involving the leg:
- the anterior tibialis muscle (Figs. 7-5, 7-6, and 7-7)

- the extensor digitorum longus muscle (Figs. 7-5, 7-6, and 7-8)
- the peroneus longus muscle (Figs. 7-5, 7-6, and 7-9)

(The approach to the proximal aspect of the peroneus longus muscle is described as part of the examination of the lateral compartment.)

*Comment:*    *Since the patellar ligament is not an active structure, as indicated by its name, it is covered in the corresponding discussion (Fig. 6-15, page 80).*

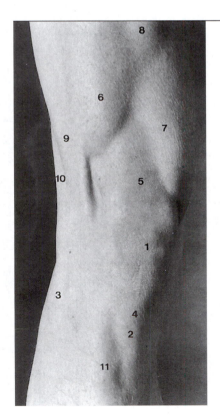

**FIGURE 7-1**
**ANTEROLATERAL VIEW OF THE KNEE**

1. Patella
2. Tibial tuberosity
3. Head of the fibula
4. Patellar ligament
5. Tendon of the quadriceps extensor muscle
6. Vastus lateralis muscle
7. Vastus medialis muscle
8. Rectus femoris muscle
9. Iliotibial band
10. Tendon of the biceps femoris muscle
11. Anterior tibialis muscle

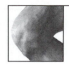

# THE THIGH

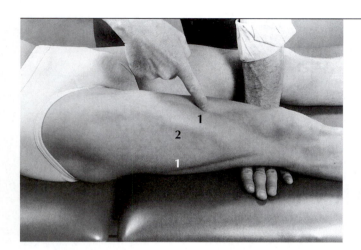

## FIGURE 7-2
### THE VASTUS LATERALIS MUSCLE

Ask the subject to apply pressure on your hand, which is placed between the popliteal fossa and the table. The vastus lateralis muscle (1) appears over the anterolateral aspect of the thigh in front and behind the iliotibial band (2).

Also see Fig. 7-3.

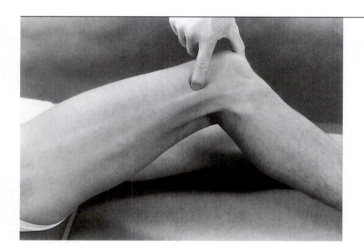

## FIGURE 7-3
### THE TENDON OF THE ILIOTIBIAL TRACT OR MAISSIAT'S BAND

With the subject's knee flexed and foot resting on the table, the band appears or is felt under your fingers over the lateral aspect of the knee as the subject begins to extend the knee. An active internal rotation of the leg accentuates its demonstration. For a better perception of this structure, the subject may also perform a complete extension of the knee (see Part II, "The Thigh," Figs. 4-15 and 4-16).

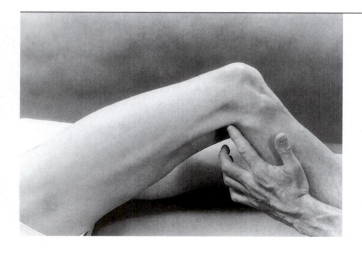

## FIGURE 7-4
### THE DISTAL ASPECT OF THE TENDON OF THE BICEPS FEMORIS MUSCLE

The essential bony landmark is the head of the fibula.

With one hand, cover the heel and resist the flexion of the knee. The other hand, placed in the area of the head of the fibula, approaches the examined structure, which constitutes the superolateral border of the popliteal fossa (see also Figs. 7-24 and 7-25).

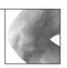

# THE LEG

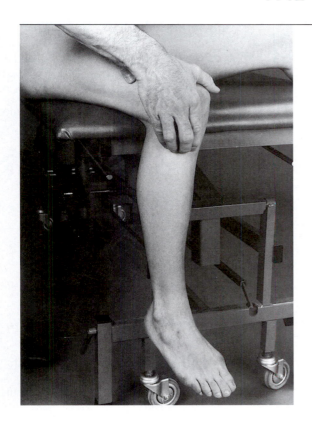

## FIGURE 7-5

### LOCALIZATION OF THE ANTERIOR TIBIALIS, EXTENSOR DIGITORUM LONGUS, AND PERONEUS LONGUS MUSCLES

The subject is sitting on the side of the table, possibly with legs crossed. The foot is in a dependent, normally relaxed position.

The subject may also be placed in supine position, but with the trunk elevated so that he or she has visual control over the movements of the foot.

Your palpating hand is positioned with a digital grip over the superolateral aspect of the leg, between the head of the fibula and the anterior tuberosity of the tibia.

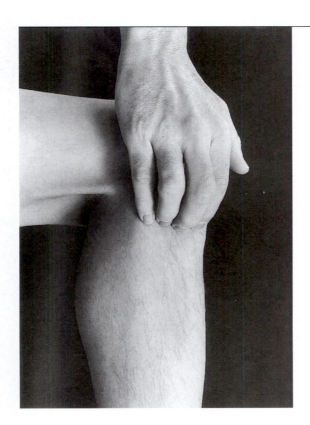

## FIGURE 7-6

### CLOSEUP ON THE LOCALIZATION DESCRIBED ABOVE

More precisely, your fifth and fourth fingers are placed against the anterior portion of the head of the fibula while the third and second fingers are positioned over the lateral border of the lateral tuberosity of the tibia, just below the oblique tibial crest and the tubercle of Gerdy (infracondylar tubercle).

With your hand in this position, your fifth finger faces the peroneus longus muscle. The fourth finger faces the extensor digitorum longus muscle, while the third and second fingers face the anterior tibialis muscle.

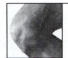

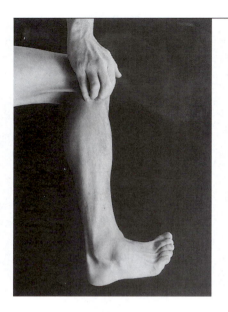

### FIGURE 7-7
### LOCALIZATION OF THE PROXIMAL ASPECT OF THE ANTERIOR TIBIALIS MUSCLE

From the starting position described in Figs. 7-5 and 7-6, the subject is asked to bring the foot into adduction, supination, and dorsiflexion—the actions of the anterior tibialis muscle.

The muscular contraction is felt beneath the fingers, more precisely under the second and third fingers.

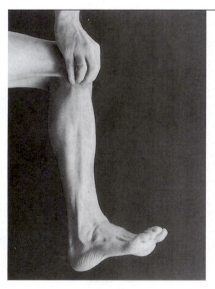

### FIGURE 7-8
### LOCALIZATION OF THE PROXIMAL ASPECT OF THE EXTENSOR DIGITORUM LONGUS MUSCLE

From the starting position described in Figs. 7-5 and 7-6, the subject is asked to bring the foot into abduction, pronation, and dorsiflexion—the actions of the extensor digitorum longus muscle.

The muscular contraction is perceived beneath the fingers, more precisely under the fourth finger.

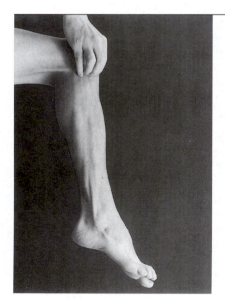

### FIGURE 7-9
### LOCALIZATION OF THE PROXIMAL ASPECT OF THE PERONEUS LONGUS MUSCLE

From the position described above, the subject is asked to bring the foot into abduction, pronation, and plantarflexion—the actions of the peroneus longus muscle.

The muscular contraction is perceived beneath the fingers, more precisely under the fourth and fifth fingers.

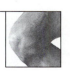

# THE ANTEROMEDIAL REGION

With the knee flexed at 90°, the muscular and tendinous structures accessible by palpation are, from below upward, as follows:

- the tendon of the semitendinosus muscle (Figs. 7-11 through 7-14)
- the tendon of the gracilis muscle (Figs. 7-11, 7-12, 7-13, and 7-15)
- the semimembranosus muscle (Fig. 7-17)

- the sartorius muscle (Figs. 7-11, 7-12, 7-13, and 7-16)
- the distal tendon of the vertical bundle of the adductor magnus muscle (Fig. 7-18)
- the muscular body of the vastus medialis muscle (Fig. 7-19)

*Comment:* **The semitendinosus, gracilis, and sartorius muscles constitute the muscles of the pes anserinus. Their approach is discussed on the next page.**

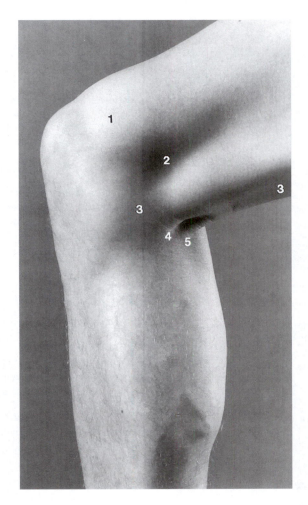

**FIGURE 7-10**
**MEDIAL VIEW OF THE KNEE**

1.  Vastus medialis muscle
2.  Tendon of the adductor magnus muscle
3.  Semimembranosus muscle
4.  Tendon of the gracilis muscle
5.  Tendon of the semitendinosus muscle

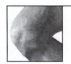

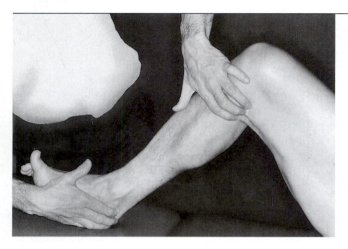

## Figure 7-11

### Localization of the muscles of the pes anserinus over the medial border of the tibia

First localize the upper end of the medial border of the tibia and position your fingers as shown in the figure. With the other hand, offer resistance to a flexion and an isometric internal rotation of the knee. The subject then proceeds with movements in a contraction-relaxation sequence to permit better perception of the tendons and their topography.

- the tendon of the semitendinosus is the most posterior and is well perceived under the index finger
- the tendon of the gracilis muscle is located just above the previous tendon and is perceived under the middle finger
- the distal aspect of the sartorius muscle overlies that of the gracilis muscle. The placement under tension of this muscle is perceived under the ring finger (see also Fig. 7-16).

*Comment:*   *If the perception of the tendons over the medial border of the tibia is difficult, a more proximal palpation should be done by moving the fingers slightly backward.*

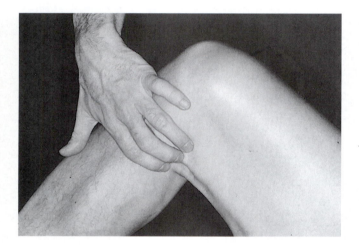

## Figure 7-12

### Closeup of the localization described above

This figure is interesting since it clearly shows the respective positions of the different tendons and muscular bodies. The index finger faces the tendon of the semitendinosus muscle. The middle finger, which is not visualized in this picture, faces the tendon of the gracilis muscle and the ring finger faces the sartorius muscle.

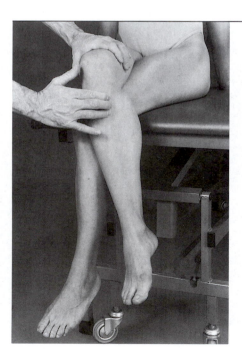

## Figure 7-13

### Localization of the placement under tension of the muscles of the pes anserinus over the anterior and medial aspects of the tibia

With a wide grip, position your fingers below the medial condyle of the tibia, covering the anterior tuberosity of the tibia in the extension of the examined tendons (Figs. 7-11 and 7-12).

The muscular action is the same as that demonstrated in Fig. 7-11. A flexion of the subject's knee, which may be carried out isometrically against the contralateral lower extremity, is associated with an internal rotation of the leg (performed by bringing the forefoot medially), since these muscles of the pes anserinus are also internal rotators of the leg. One then perceives through the skin the placement of the pes anserinus muscles under tension.

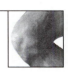

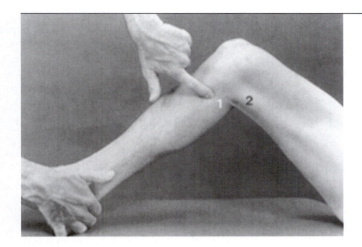

## FIGURE 7-14
### THE DISTAL TENDON OF THE SEMITENDINOSUS MUSCLE

The essential bony landmark is the superior end of the medial border of the tibia.

With the knee flexed at approximately 90°, your one hand, positioned against the medial aspect of the foot, offers resistance to the flexion and internal rotation of the knee, while the other hand slides up along the medial border of the tibia until it meets the investigated tendon (1).

The subject may also be asked to press his or her heel against the table, thereby performing an isometric contraction of the knee flexion, and to carry out rapid, consecutive internal rotations of the leg. Your two hands are then free for the examination.

Difficulty of approach: The localization of this tendon is reasonably easy in the male subject but much more difficult in the female in view of the presence of adipose tissue. In this case, if any difficulty is encountered, it should be investigated more posteriorly in the soft tissues of the upper calf or at the level of the popliteal fossa (see Fig. 7-21).

### FIGURES 7-14 AND 7-15

1.   Semitendinosus muscle
2.   Gracilis muscle

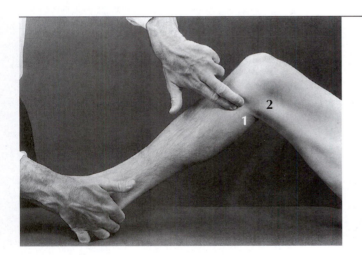

## FIGURE 7-15
### THE DISTAL TENDON OF THE GRACILIS MUSCLE

The bony landmark—the medial border of the tibia—remains the same, and this is where your fingers should be placed. Your other hand offers resistance to the flexion and internal rotation of the knee by covering the heel and applying the forearm against the medial border of the foot.

The investigated tendon (2) (see also Fig. 7-22) is perceived above the tendon of the semitendinosus muscle and below the sartorius muscle (see also Fig. 7-16), which may cover it partially.

Difficulty of approach: The comment is the same as that made for the tendon of the semitendinosus muscle (Fig. 7-14).

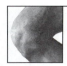

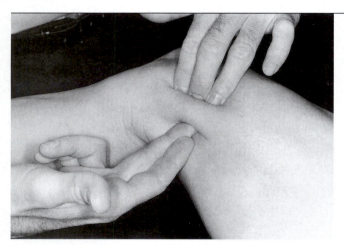

**FIGURE 7-16**
**DISTAL ASPECT OF THE SARTORIUS MUSCLE: MEDIAL VIEW, KNEE SEMIFLEXED**

The subject's knee should be placed in almost complete extension and the hip in slight external rotation in order to have the muscular body appear over the medial aspect of the knee.

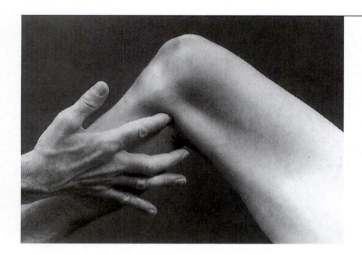

**FIGURE 7-17**
**THE TENDON OF THE SEMIMEMBRANOSUS MUSCLE**

The essential bony landmark is formed by the junction of the medial and posterior surfaces of the medial condyle of the tibia. Position the leg in external rotation in order to demonstrate this bony structure. Your hand offers resistance to the flexion and internal rotation of the knee. The other hand looks for the tendon presenting under the fingers as a full, relatively thick cylindrical cord.

More anteriorly, the reflected tendon of this muscle slides under the horizontal tibial ligament of the tibia's internal tuberosity.

Difficulty of approach: There is none if one remembers to position the leg properly in external rotation, thereby clearing out this tendon.

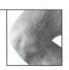

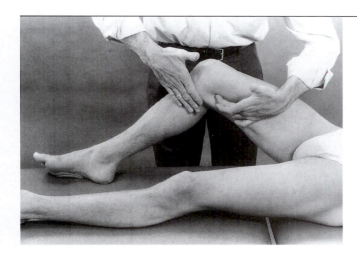

## FIGURE 7-18

### THE DISTAL TENDON OF THE VERTICAL BUNDLE OF THE ADDUCTOR MAGNUS MUSCLE—ALSO CALLED INFERIOR BUNDLE OR INTERNAL PORTION OF THE ADDUCTOR MAGNUS MUSCLE

The essential bony landmark is the adductor tubercle (see also Fig. 5-21).

The essential muscular landmark is the vastus medialis muscle (see Fig. 7-19).

The investigated tendon is located behind this muscle. It presents beneath the fingers as a full and relatively thick cylindrical cord (see also Part II, "The Thigh," Fig. 4-23).

*Comment:* *Your distal hand may be placed against the medial aspect of the knee, pushing laterally in the direction of the abduction of the hip, while the subject is asked to resist this movement. The tendon will be better perceived under the fingers.*

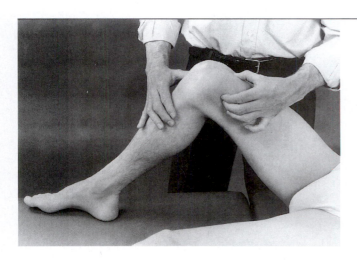

## FIGURE 7-19

### THE MUSCULAR BODY OF THE VASTUS MEDIALIS MUSCLE

To make this muscle prominent if the knee is flexed, ask the subject to press his or her heel against the ground or the table.

If the knee is in extension, ask for a contraction of the quadriceps extensor muscle.

In relation to the patella, the muscular body is demonstrated superiorly and medially.

*Comment:* *Note the lower position of this muscle as compared with that of the vastus lateralis muscle (Fig. 7-1) (see also Part II, "The Thigh," Fig. 4-10).*

# THE POSTERIOR REGION

The muscular and tendinous structures accessible by palpation are as follows below.

At the level of the thigh:

- the tendon of the semitendinosus muscle (Fig. 7-21)
- the tendon of the gracilis muscle (Fig. 7-22)
- the semimembranosus muscle (Fig. 7-23)
- the tendon of the biceps femoris muscle (Fig. 7-24)
- the biceps femoris muscle—short head (see Fig. 7-25)

At the level of the leg:

- the medial head of the gastrocnemius muscle (see Part IV, "The Leg")
- the lateral head of the gastrocnemius muscle (see Part IV, "The Leg")

*Comment:* *In this part, we discuss only the muscles located at the level of the thigh as well as the tendon of the popliteus muscle. For the other muscles, refer to Part IV, "The Leg."*

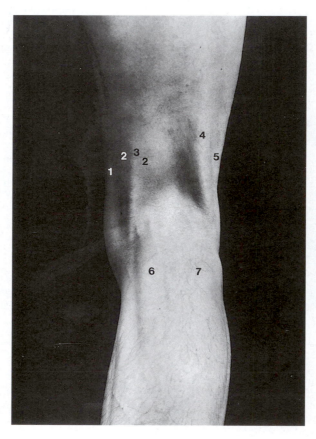

**FIGURE 7-20**
**POSTERIOR VIEW OF THE KNEE**

1. Gracilis muscle
2. Semimembranosus muscle
3. Semitendinosus muscle
4. Biceps femoris muscle
5. Iliotibial band
6. Medial head of the gastrocnemius muscle
7. Lateral head of the gastrocnemius muscle

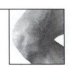

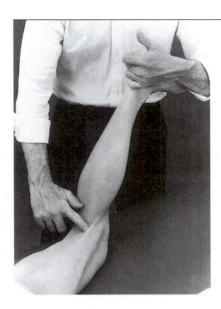

### FIGURE 7-21
### TENDON OF THE SEMITENDINOSUS MUSCLE

With the subject prone, wrap your distal hand around the heel and offer resistance to the flexion of the knee. Resistance may also be offered to the internal rotation of the knee (then your forearm is placed against the medial border of the foot).

The tendon of the semitendinosus muscle is the most posterior and lateral of the musculotendinous structures demonstrated over the posteromedial aspect of the thigh.

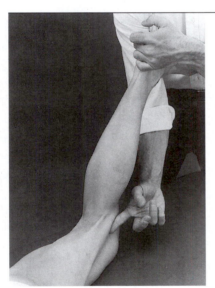

### FIGURE 7-22
### THE TENDON OF THE GRACILIS MUSCLE

The subject's position and the resistance offered are the same as described in Fig. 7-21.

The tendon of the gracilis muscle is demonstrated anterior and medial to the tendon of the semitendinosus muscle.

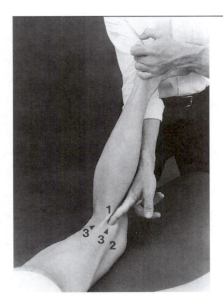

### FIGURE 7-23
### THE SEMIMEMBRANOSUS MUSCLE

The subject's position as well as the resistance offered are the same as those described in Fig. 7-21.

The semimembranosus muscle (3) is a muscular body perceived beneath the fingers between the tendons of the semitendinosus (1) and gracilis (2) muscles. It is also palpated lateral to the tendon of the semitendinosus muscle (1).

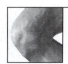

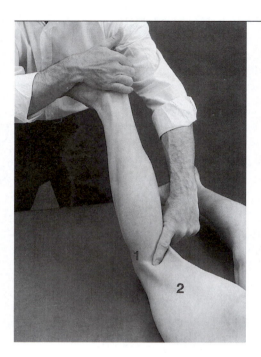

### FIGURE 7-24
#### LOCALIZATION OF THE TENDON OF THE BICEPS FEMORIS MUSCLE IN THE POPLITEAL FOSSA

With the subject prone, cover the heel with one hand and place your forearm against the lateral border of the foot in order to resist a flexion and an external rotation of the knee simultaneously. The tendon is demonstrated (see figure) (1) in the posterolateral portion of the popliteal fossa. The muscular body (2) of the biceps femoris muscle is also visible (see figure).

1. Tendon of the biceps femoris muscle inserting into the head of the fibula
2. Muscular body of the long head of the biceps femoris muscle

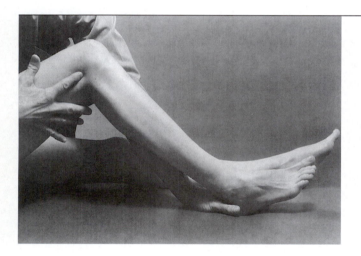

### FIGURE 7-25
#### THE TENDON OF THE POPLITEUS MUSCLE

While your one hand offers resistance to the flexion of the knee, the other is placed behind the fibular collateral ligament (see also Figs. 6-2 and 6-3).

The investigated tendon is palpated just behind the latter structure. Its palpation is not obvious in all subjects.

# NERVES AND VESSELS

**8**

---

## THE POPLITEAL FOSSA

The neurovascular structures accessible by palpation are as follows:

- the tibial nerve (Figs. 8-3 and 8-5)
- the common peroneal nerve (Fig. 8-7)

- the sural nerve (or sural) (Fig. 8-8)
- the popliteal artery (Figs. 8-10, 8-11, and 8-12)

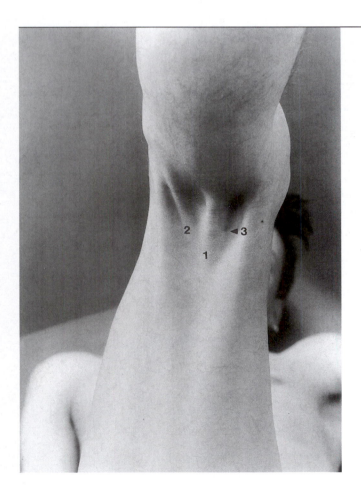

**FIGURE 8-1**
**POSTERIOR VIEW OF THE POPLITEAL FOSSA. POSITION OF THE SUBJECT: DORSAL DECUBITUS, HIP AND KNEE FLEXED**

1. Tibial nerve
2. Common peroneal nerve
3. Popliteal artery

*Comment:*     ***The arrowhead indicates the landmark for an optimal approach to the popliteal artery.***

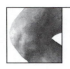 

# THE TIBIAL NERVE

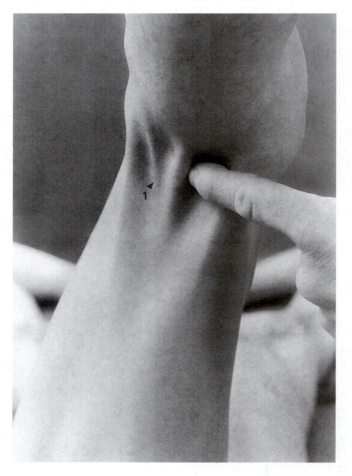

**FIGURE 8-2**
**POSTERIOR VIEW OF THE POPLITEAL FOSSA. POSITION OF THE SUBJECT: SUPINE, HIP AND KNEE FLEXED**

The index finger indicates the tibial nerve.

1. Common peroneal nerve

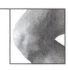

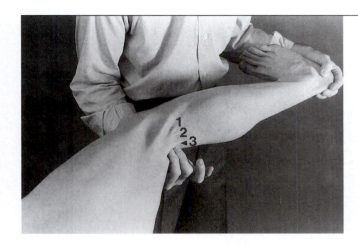

## FIGURE 8-3
### DEMONSTRATION OF THE TIBIAL NERVE IN SIDE LYING

The subject is in side-lying position. The hip is flexed beyond 90°, the knee is slightly flexed, and the ankle is also placed in dorsiflexion.

The index finger indicates the investigated structure.

---

### FIGURES 8-3 AND 8-4

1. Common peroneal nerve
2. Sural nerve
3. Tibial nerve

---

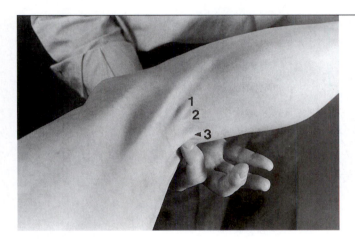

## FIGURE 8-4
### CLOSEUP VIEW OF THE POPLITEAL FOSSA

The technique of demonstration is the same as that described above. The subject is placed in side-lying position, the ankle is brought into complete dorsiflexion, the knee is slightly flexed, and the hip is progressively brought in more or less complete flexion.

If this is not sufficient to demonstrate the nerve in the middle of the popliteal fossa, the subject should be asked to flex the upper body (Fig. 8-5).

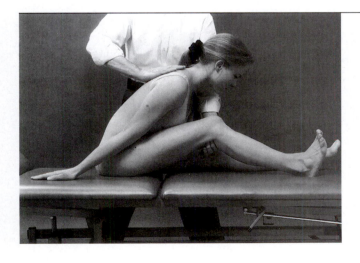

## FIGURE 8-5
### DEMONSTRATION OF THE TIBIAL NERVE

With the knee in flexion between 90 and 45°, the subject brings the ankle into maximal dorsiflexion. The palpating hand should be positioned in the center of the popliteal fossa. The other hand, placed on the subject's back, supports a flexion of the upper body in order to place the sciatic nerve and its terminal branches, including the tibial nerve, under more tension and to make them more accessible to examination.

The investigated nerve is palpated as a full cylindrical cord.

# THE PERONEAL NERVE

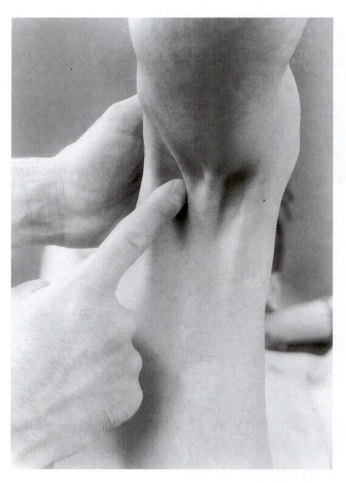

**FIGURE 8-6**
**POSTERIOR VIEW OF THE POPLITEAL FOSSA. SUBJECT'S**
**POSITION: SUPINE, HIP AND KNEE FLEXED**

The index finger indicates the peroneal nerve.

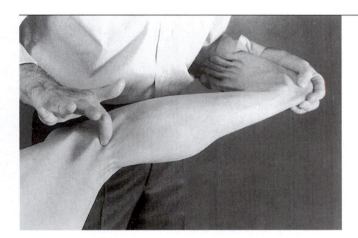

## FIGURE 8-7
### DEMONSTRATION OF THE PERONEAL NERVE

The technique of demonstration is the same as that described for the tibial nerve.

The index finger indicates the investigated structure.

# THE SURAL NERVE

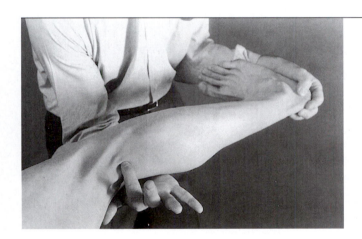

## FIGURE 8-8
### DEMONSTRATION OF THE ACCESSORY/SUBORDINATE EXTERNAL SURAL NERVE

The technique of demonstration is the same as that described for the tibial nerve.

The index finger indicates the investigated structure.

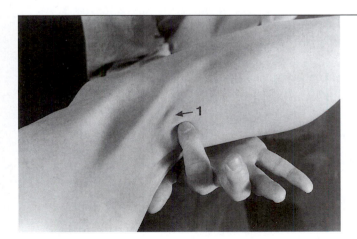

## FIGURE 8-9
### CLOSEUP ON THE POPLITEAL FOSSA

With regard to the technique of demonstration, see Figs. 8-2 and 8-4.

The index finger indicates the investigated structure, i.e., the external saphenous or sural nerve. Laterally, the peroneal nerve (1) is seen as it passes toward the neck of the fibula.

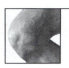

# THE POPLITEAL ARTERY

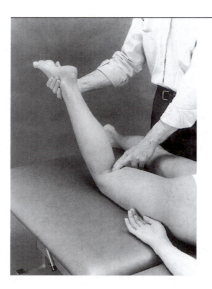

**FIGURE 8-10**

**PULSE EXAMINATION IN THE POPLITEAL FOSSA. STEP 1**

The knee is brought into more or less complete extension. By leaning on the tendon of the semitendinosus muscle, you can apply a two- or three-finger grip in the superomedial aspect of the popliteal fossa.

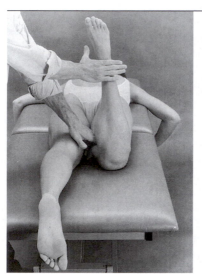

**FIGURE 8-11**

**PULSE EXAMINATION IN THE POPLITEAL FOSSA. STEP 2**

As you look for the popliteal pulse, which is found in proximity to the tibial nerve, the subject's knee is progressively brought into flexion and your digital grip is directed toward the central portion of the popliteal fossa.

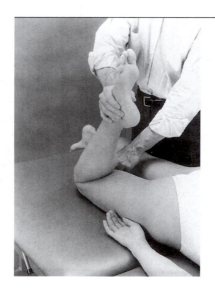

**FIGURE 8-12**

**PULSE EXAMINATION IN THE POPLITEAL FOSSA. STEP 3**

Knee positioning in more or less maximal flexion allows an optimal relaxation of the posterior fibrous plane of the knee. Access to the popliteal artery is facilitated, and it is palpated over the medial aspect of the tibial nerve.

# THE LEG

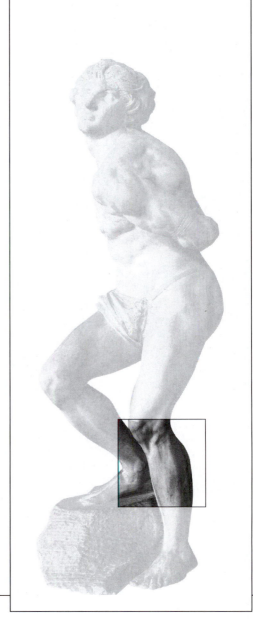

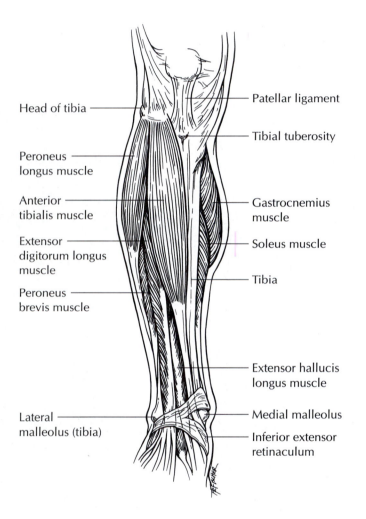

Head of tibia

Peroneus longus muscle

Anterior tibialis muscle

Extensor digitorum longus muscle

Peroneus brevis muscle

Lateral malleolus (tibia)

Patellar ligament

Tibial tuberosity

Gastrocnemius muscle

Soleus muscle

Tibia

Extensor hallucis longus muscle

Medial malleolus

Inferior extensor retinaculum

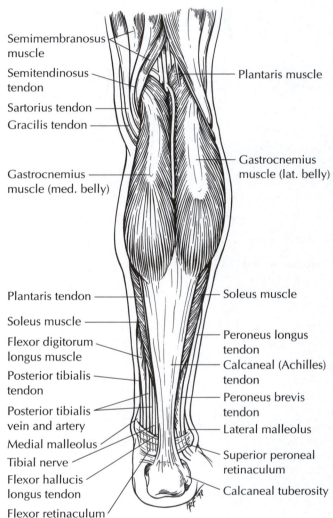

Semimembranosus muscle

Semitendinosus tendon

Sartorius tendon

Gracilis tendon

Gastrocnemius muscle (med. belly)

Plantaris tendon

Soleus muscle

Flexor digitorum longus muscle

Posterior tibialis tendon

Posterior tibialis vein and artery

Medial malleolus

Tibial nerve

Flexor hallucis longus tendon

Flexor retinaculum

Plantaris muscle

Gastrocnemius muscle (lat. belly)

Soleus muscle

Peroneus longus tendon

Calcaneal (Achilles) tendon

Peroneus brevis tendon

Lateral malleolus

Superior peroneal retinaculum

Calcaneal tuberosity

# ILLUSTRATED STUDY OF THE LOWER LEG (LATERAL)

# ILLUSTRATED STUDY OF THE LOWER LEG (MEDIAL)

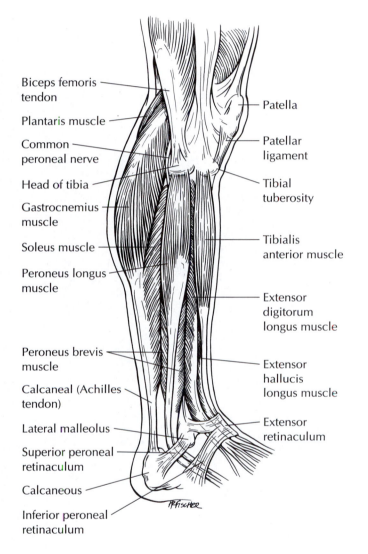

Biceps femoris tendon

Plantaris muscle

Common peroneal nerve

Head of tibia

Gastrocnemius muscle

Soleus muscle

Peroneus longus muscle

Peroneus brevis muscle

Calcaneal (Achilles) tendon)

Lateral malleolus

Superior peroneal retinaculum

Calcaneous

Inferior peroneal retinaculum

Patella

Patellar ligament

Tibial tuberosity

Tibialis anterior muscle

Extensor digitorum longus muscle

Extensor hallucis longus muscle

Extensor retinaculum

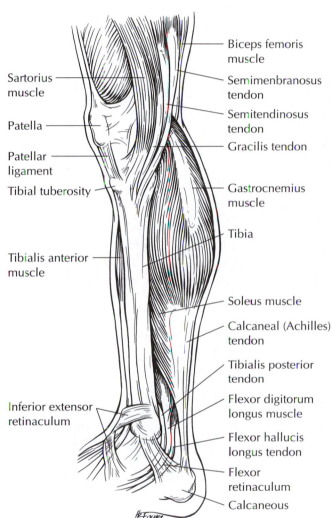

Sartorius muscle

Patella

Patellar ligament

Tibial tuberosity

Tibialis anterior muscle

Inferior extensor retinaculum

Biceps femoris muscle

Semimenbranosus tendon

Semitendinosus tendon

Gracilis tendon

Gastrocnemius muscle

Tibia

Soleus muscle

Calcaneal (Achilles) tendon

Tibialis posterior tendon

Flexor digitorum longus muscle

Flexor hallucis longus tendon

Flexor retinaculum

Calcaneous

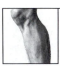

# TOPOGRAPHIC PRESENTATION OF THE LEG

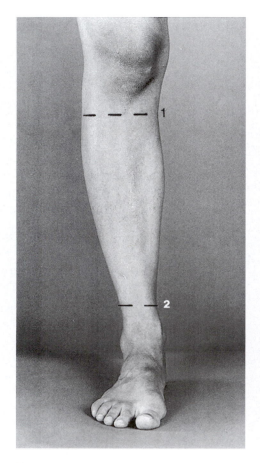

**FIGURE 9-1**
**ANTERIOR VIEW**

1. Superior border

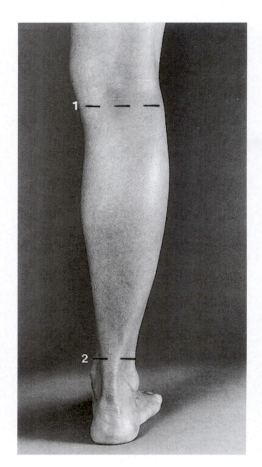

**FIGURE 9-2**
**POSTERIOR VIEW**

2. Inferior border

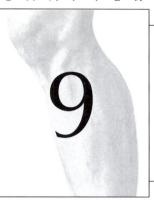
# OSTEOLOGY

## LEG

The bony structures accessible by palpation are

- the tibia
  —the anterior border (Fig. 9-3)
  —the medial border (Fig. 9-4)

  —the medial surface (Fig. 9-5)
  —the posterior surface (Fig. 9-6)
- the fibula
  —the lateral surface (Fig. 9-7)

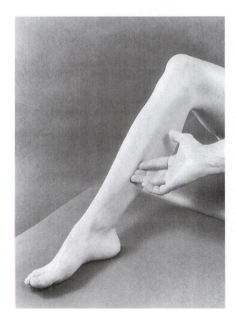

**FIGURE 9-3**
**THE ANTERIOR BORDER OF THE TIBIA**

This border extends from the tibial tuberosity down to the medial malleolus.

In its superior three-quarters, it has the shape of a fish bone and it is called the *crest of the tibia.*

In its inferior quarter, the border deviates medially toward the medial malleolus and becomes rounded.

Directly under the skin, the anterior border is entirely accessible.

**FIGURE 9-4**
**THE MEDIAL BORDER OF THE TIBIA**

Extending from the medial condyle of the tibia down to the medial malleolus, this structure borders medially the medial surface of the tibial shaft. It is also entirely accessible for investigation.

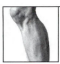

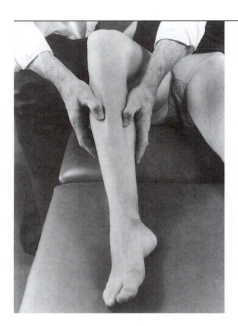

### FIGURE 9-5
#### THE MEDIAL SURFACE OF THE TIBIA

This area has a smooth, flat surface which is in direct contact with the skin throughout its length.

Very close to the anterior tuberosity of the tibia, the muscles of the pes anserinus insert into the proximal portion of this surface.

Located between the anterior border (Fig. 9-3) and the medial border (Fig. 9-4), it is entirely accessible for investigation.

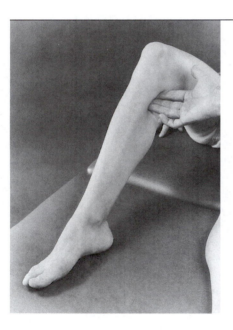

### FIGURE 9-6
#### THE POSTERIOR SURFACE OF THE TIBIA

This area is partially accessible for investigation, behind the medial border of the tibia, particularly at the proximal and distal ends of the tibial shaft.

In this figure, the leg is positioned in external rotation in order to expose the posterior surface of the tibia, palpated behind the proximal aspect of its medial border (see also Fig. 9-4). Care must be taken to relax the posterior muscles of the leg significantly.

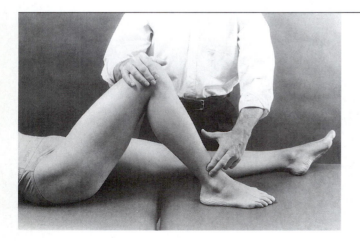

### FIGURE 9-7
#### THE LATERAL SURFACE OF THE FIBULA

This surface is directly accessible in its distal part. The distal end is covered by an oblique crest extending downward and backward, dividing it in two parts:

- an anterior part, triangular in shape, directly subcutaneous and accessible without difficulty
- a posterior part, over which the tendons of the lateral peroneal muscles (peroneus longus and peroneus brevis muscles) slide

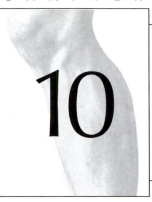

# 10

# MYOLOGY

## THE ANTERIOR MUSCULAR GROUP

The anterior muscular group includes these four muscles:

- the anterior tibialis muscle (Figs. 10-2 through 10-5)
- the extensor hallucis longus muscle (Figs. 10-8, 10-9, and 10-10)
- the extensor digitorum longus muscle (Figs. 10-11 and 10-12)
- the peroneus tertius muscle (Fig. 10-13)

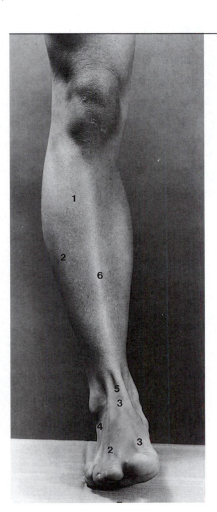

**FIGURE 10-1**
**ANTERIOR VIEW OF THE LEG**

1. Anterior tibialis muscle
2. Extensor digitorum longus muscle
3. Extensor hallucis longus muscle
4. Peroneus tertius muscle
5. Extensor retinaculum
6. Anterior border of the tibia

# THE ANTERIOR TIBIALIS MUSCLE

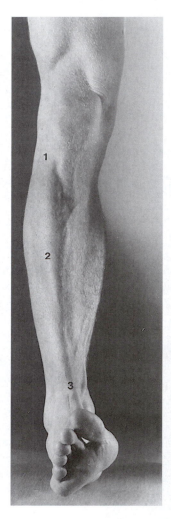

**FIGURE 10-2**
**ANTERIOR VIEW OF THE LEG**

1. Anterior tibialis muscle—proximal insertion
2. Anterior tibialis muscle—muscular body
3. Anterior tibialis muscle—distal tendon

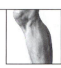

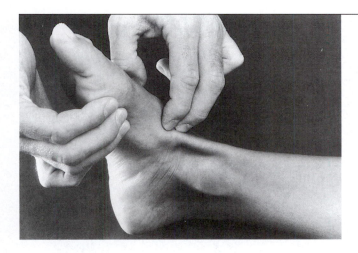

## FIGURE 10-3

### THE DISTAL PORTION OF THE TENDON OF THE ANTERIOR TIBIALIS MUSCLE

After bringing the foot into adduction, supination, and dorsiflexion, resist this muscular action by placing a digital grip positioned over the medial border of the foot in order to demonstrate the tendon. This tendon is the most medial of the tendons of the proximal foot and is located just in front of the medial malleolus.

In this figure, the digital grip faces the tendon, close to its distal insertion into the anteroinferior aspect of the medial surface of the medial cuneiform bone. This insertion extends into the inferomedial aspect of the base of the first metatarsal bone.

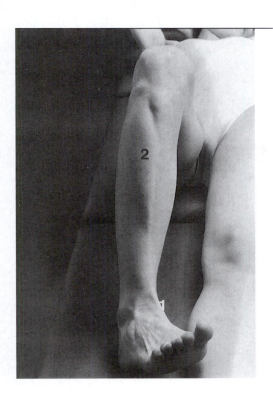

## FIGURE 10-4

### THE ANTERIOR TIBIALIS MUSCLE IN THE LEG

The tendon (1) follows the lateral aspect of the tibial crest or of the anterior border of the tibia. It extends as a muscular body (2), which is also lateral to the tibial crest and medial to the extensor digitorum longus muscle.

The requested muscular action is the same as that described above.

*Comment:    In this picture, the muscle is easily demonstrated.*

1.   Tendon of the anterior tibialis muscle
2.   Muscular body of the anterior tibialis muscle.

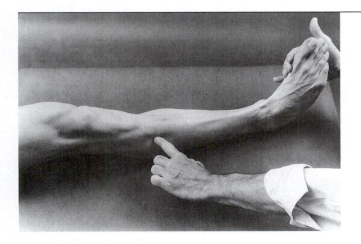

## FIGURE 10-5

### PROXIMAL INSERTION OF THE ANTERIOR TIBIALIS MUSCLE

Also see Part III, "The Knee" (Figs. 7-5, 7-6, and 7-7).

Obtain the same foot positioning as that described in Fig. 10-3. The resistance is also applied against the medial border of the foot in order to clearly note the muscular body as it tightens under the fingers.

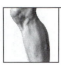
# THE EXTRINSIC EXTENSOR MUSCLES OF THE TOES AND THE PERONEUS TERTIUS MUSCLE

This group includes three muscles:

- the extensor hallucis longus muscle (Figs. 10-8, 10-9, and 10-10)
- the extensor digitorum longus muscle (Figs. 10-11 and 10-12)
- the peroneus tertius muscle (Fig. 10-13)

This last muscle, which is not consistent, extends from the inferior third of the fibula to the fifth metatarsal bone.

*Comment:*    *The extensor digitorum brevis muscle also participates in the extension of the toes, but it is an intrinsic muscle of the foot, and is discussed in Part V, "The Ankle and Foot."*

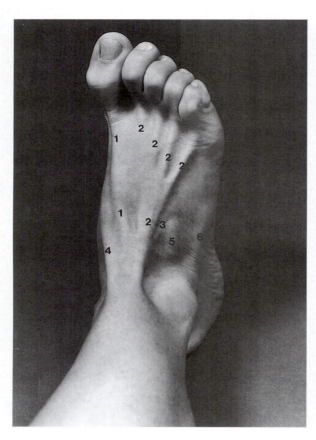

**FIGURE 10-6**
**DORSAL VIEW OF THE FOOT**

1. Extensor hallucis longus muscle
2. Extensor digitorum longus muscle
3. Peroneus tertius muscle
4. Anterior tibialis muscle
5. Extensor hallucis brevis muscle
6. Peroneus brevis muscle

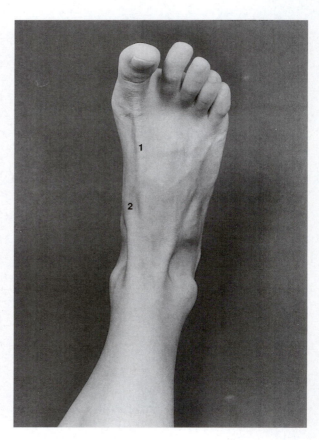

**FIGURE 10-7**
**ANTERIOR VIEW OF THE ANKLE**

1. Extensor hallucis longus muscle
2. Anterior tibialis muscle

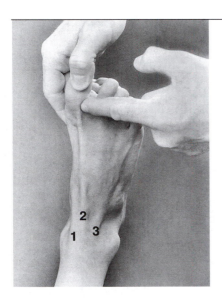

### FIGURE 10-8

#### THE TENDON OF THE EXTENSOR HALLUCIS LONGUS MUSCLE NEAR ITS DISTAL INSERTION

The subject is asked to perform a complete extension of the first toe. A resistance is applied by the examiner's thumb against the dorsal aspect of the distal phalanx of the first toe, attempting to bring it in flexion.

The index finger shows the tendon near its distal sites of insertion into the base of the dorsal aspect of the distal phalanx of the first toe as well as into the medial and lateral aspects of the base of the proximal phalanx.

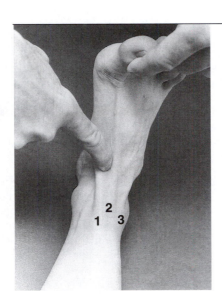

### FIGURE 10-9

#### THE TENDON OF THE EXTENSOR HALLUCIS LONGUS MUSCLE IN THE PROXIMAL FOOT (OR "HINDFOOT")

The requested muscular action is the same as that described above.

The index finger shows the tendon as it passes through the proximal aspect of the foot.

---

#### FIGURES **10-8, 10-9,** AND **10-10**

1. Anterior tibialis muscle
2. Extensor hallucis longus muscle
3. Extensor digitorum longus muscle

---

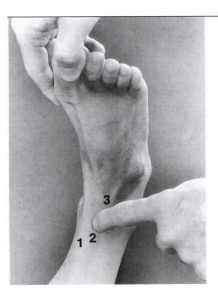

### FIGURE 10-10

#### THE MUSCULAR BODY OF THE EXTENSOR HALLUCIS LONGUS MUSCLE OVER THE DISTAL ASPECT OF THE LEG

The tendon slides behind the extensor retinaculum and joins a muscular body located proximally between the anterior tibialis muscle medially and the extensor digitorum longus muscle laterally.

To better visualize the position of the investigated muscle, consult the figures demonstrating these two muscles (pages 107 and 110, respectively).

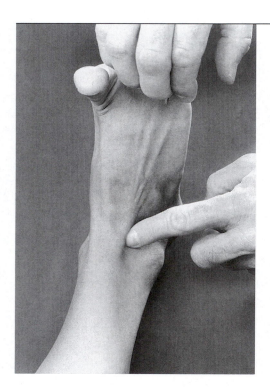

**FIGURE 10-11**

**THE TENDONS OF THE EXTENSOR DIGITORUM LONGUS MUSCLE**

The distal hand is positioned as shown here in order to resist an extension of the toes. It is useful to ask the subject to maintain an active dorsiflexion, abduction, and pronation of the foot (these last two movements are not demonstrated in this figure).

Each of the tendons leading to the four toes must be followed from its distal end up to the proximal foot. In this picture, the tendon is approached at the level of the proximal foot.

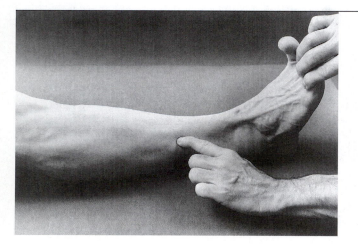

**FIGURE 10-12**

**THE EXTENSOR DIGITORUM LONGUS MUSCLE AT THE LEVEL OF THE DISTAL LEG**

The muscular body, which follows the tendon, lies throughout the length of the leg and is located, from above downward, between the peroneus longus and peroneus brevis muscles laterally, and the anterior tibialis muscle medially. The latter muscles are located through their actions. This allows a better localization of the investigated muscular body (see also Fig. 10-15).

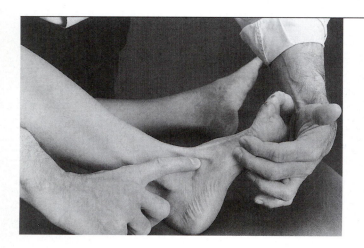

**FIGURE 10-13**

**THE PERONEUS TERTIUS MUSCLE**

This structure appears as a tendon over the lateral aspect of the tendon of the extensor digitorum longus muscle, leading to the fifth toe.

To make this muscle prominent, the subject is asked to invert the foot with or without resistance. The tendon extends toward the dorsal surface of the base of the fifth metatarsal bone.

# THE LATERAL MUSCULAR GROUP

This group includes two muscles:

- the peroneus longus muscle (Figs. 10-16, 10-17, and 10-18)

- the peroneus brevis muscle (Figs. 10-20, 10-21, and 10-22)

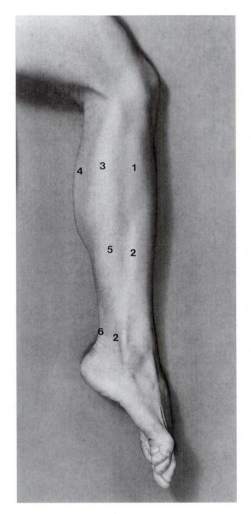

**FIGURE 10-14**
**LATERAL VIEW OF THE LEG**

1.  Peroneus longus muscle
2.  Peroneus brevis muscle
3.  Lateral head of the gastrocnemius muscle
4.  Medial head of the gastrocnemius muscle
5.  Soleus muscle
6.  Achilles tendon

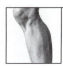

# THE PERONEUS LONGUS MUSCLE

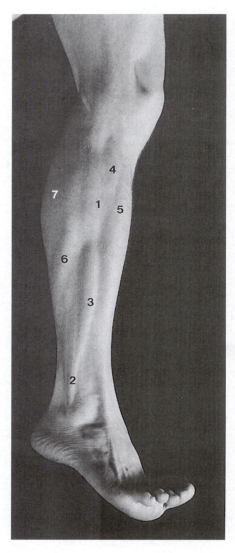

**FIGURE 10-15**
**LATERAL VIEW OF THE LEG**

1. Peroneus longus muscle
2. Tendon of the peroneus longus muscle
3. Peroneus brevis muscle
4. Extensor digitorum longus muscle
5. Anterior tibialis muscle
6. Soleus muscle
7. Lateral head of the gastrocnemius muscle

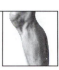

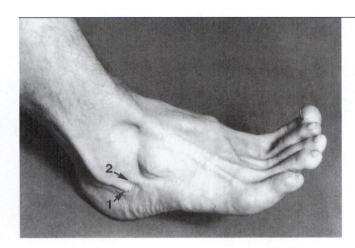

## FIGURE 10-16

### THE TENDON OF THE PERONEUS LONGUS MUSCLE AT THE LATERAL BORDER OF THE FOOT

The subject is asked to position the foot in abduction. After passing around the lateral malleolus, the tendon (1) slides against the lateral surface of the calcaneum, passes behind the peroneal tubercle (2), and enters the lateral border of the foot in the peroneal groove of the cuboid bone.

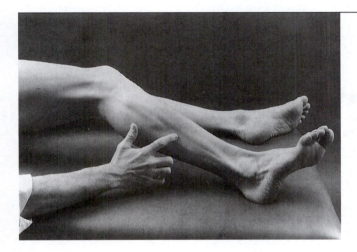

## FIGURE 10-17

### TENDON OF THE PERONEUS LONGUS MUSCLE AT THE LEVEL OF THE LEG

The muscular action is identical to that described above. At this level, the tendon is located at approximately the middle aspect of the lateral surface of the leg. It lies against the muscular body of the peroneus brevis muscle, which extends beyond it anteriorly and posteriorly (see Fig. 10-22).

### FIGURES 10-17 AND 10-18

1.  Peroneus longus muscle
2.  Peroneus brevis muscle
3.  Extensor digitorum longus muscle
4.  Soleus muscle

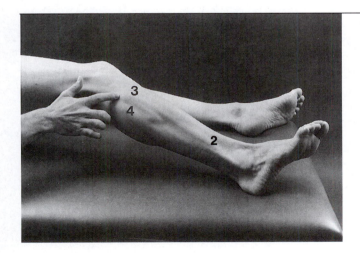

## FIGURE 10-18

### THE MUSCULAR BODY OF THE PERONEUS LONGUS MUSCLE

The muscular action is the same as that described above (Fig. 10-16).

The muscular body is located in the superior portion of the lateral surface of the leg, between the extensor digitorum longus muscle (3) anteriorly and the soleus muscle (4) posteriorly.

# THE PERONEUS BREVIS MUSCLE

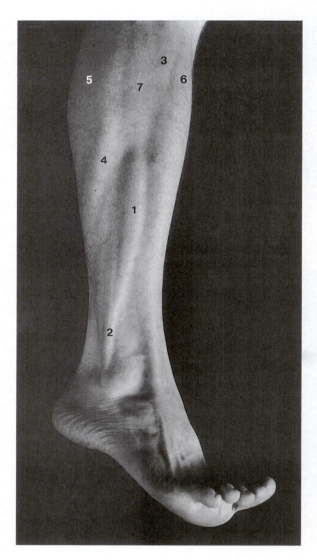

**FIGURE 10-19**
**LATERAL VIEW OF THE INFERIOR TWO-THIRDS OF THE LEG**

1.  Peroneus brevis muscle
2.  Tendon of the peroneus longus muscle
3.  Extensor digitorum longus muscle
4.  Soleus muscle
5.  Lateral head of the gastrocnemius muscle
6.  Anterior tibialis muscle
7.  Peroneus longus muscle

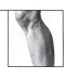

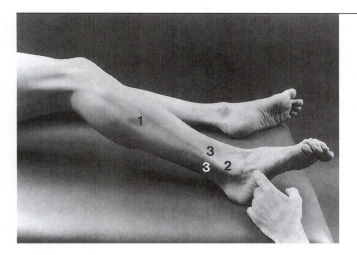

## Figure 10-20

### The tendon of the peroneus brevis muscle in its most distal course over the lateral border of the foot

A movement of pure abduction at the level of the foot is sufficient to make this tendon prominent. Its course should be followed over the lateral border of the foot down to its insertion into the tuberosity of the fifth metatarsal.

*Comment:* *To visualize well its passage over the lateral surface of the calcaneum, above and in front of the peroneal tubercle, consult Part V, "The Ankle and Foot."*

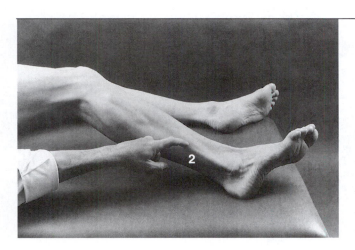

## Figure 10-21

### The peroneus brevis muscle at the level of the distal leg

The movement requested is the same as that described above. The muscular body appears in front of the tendon of the peroneus longus muscle. Movements in a contraction-relaxation sequence can improve perception of the position of the relaxed muscle.

| Figures 10-20, 10-21, and 10-22 |
| --- |
| 1. Peroneus longus muscle |
| 2. Tendon of the peroneus longus muscle |
| 3. Peroneus brevis muscle |

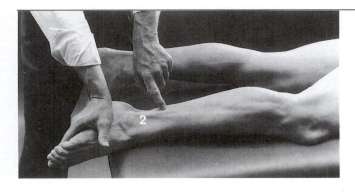

## Figure 10-22

### The peroneus brevis muscle at the leg level

The movement requested is the same as that described above. A plantarflexion of the foot may be added to improve perception of the contraction.

The muscular body is also perceived behind the tendon of the peroneus longus muscle.

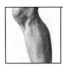

# THE POSTERIOR MUSCULAR GROUP

This group includes the following:

The superficial plane, composed of

- The triceps surae muscle, formed by:
  —the soleus muscle (Figs. 10-29, 10-30, and 10-31)
  —the medial head of the gastrocnemius muscle (Figs. 10-25 and 10-26)
  —the lateral head of the gastrocnemius muscle (Figs. 10-26 and 10-28)
- the plantaris muscle (Fig. 10-33)

The deep plane, composed of

- the popliteus muscle (Fig. 10-28)
- the posterior tibialis muscle (Figs. 10-35, 10-36, and 10-37)
- the flexor digitorum longus muscle (Figs. 10-39, 10-40, and 10-41)
- the flexor hallucis longus muscle (Figs. 10-43, 10-44, and 10-45)

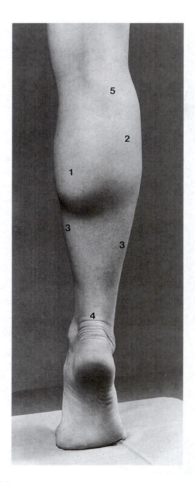

**Figure 10-23**
**Posterior view of the leg**

1. Medial head of the gastrocnemius muscle
2. Lateral head of the gastrocnemius muscle
3. Soleus muscle
4. Achilles tendon
5. Plantaris muscle

# THE SUPERFICIAL PLANE
## THE TRICEPS SURAE MUSCLE AND THE PLANTARIS MUSCLE

- The triceps surae muscle is formed by three muscles:
    —the medial head of the gastrocnemius muscle (Figs. 10-25 and 10-26)
    —the lateral head of the gastrocnemius muscle (Figs. 10-27 and 10-28)
    —the soleus muscle (Figs. 10-29, 10-30, and 10-31)

These three muscles insert distally into the calcaneum by a common tendon, the Achilles tendon (Fig. 10-32).

- The plantaris muscle (Fig. 10-33)

*Comment:* *For didactic reasons, the gastrocnemius muscle, the soleus muscle, and the plantaris muscle are studied separately and in that order.*

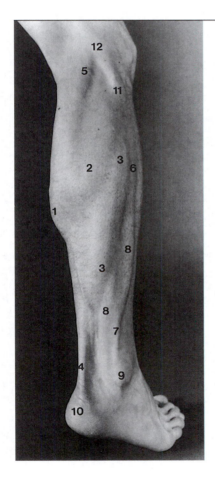

**FIGURE 10-24**
**POSTEROLATERAL VIEW OF THE LEG**

1. Medial head of the gastrocnemius muscle
2. Lateral head of the gastrocnemius muscle
3. Soleus muscle
4. Achilles tendon
5. Plantaris muscle
6. Peroneus longus muscle
7. Tendon of the peroneus longus muscle
8. Peroneus brevis muscle
9. Lateral malleolus
10. Posterior surface of the calcaneum
11. Head of the fibula
12. Tendon of the biceps femoris muscle

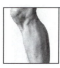

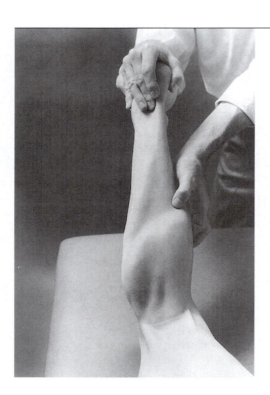

## FIGURE 10-25
### THE MEDIAL HEAD OF THE GASTROCNEMIUS MUSCLE AT THE LEG LEVEL

With your forearm leaning on the plantar aspect of the foot, the distal hand grip allows use of the "contraction-relaxation" technique by prompting plantarflexion of the ankle. With your hand covering the calcaneum, you may also offer resistance to the flexion of the knee. These two muscular actions are those of the examined muscle, which is found over the posteromedial aspect of the leg, behind the soleus muscle.

Comment:    *The muscular body of the medial head of the gastrocnemius muscle extends more inferiorly than the lateral head of the gastrocnemius muscle.*

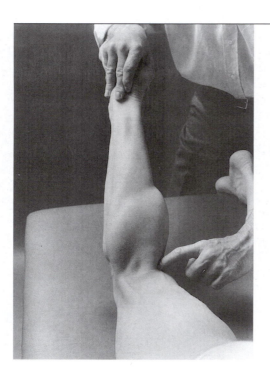

## FIGURE 10-26
### THE MEDIAL HEAD OF THE GASTROCNEMIUS MUSCLE AT THE KNEE LEVEL

The technique of placement under tension is the same as that described above.

Its proximal aspect is attached, among other structures, to the medial condylar capsule of the femur, which is only a reinforcement of the articular capsule of the knee over the posterior surface of the medial condyle of the femur. It is, therefore, approachable over the medial portion of the popliteal fossa, forming its inferomedial border.

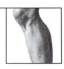

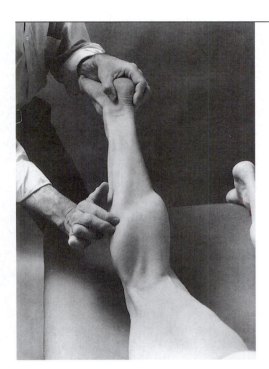

## FIGURE 10-27

### THE LATERAL HEAD OF THE GASTROCNEMIUS MUSCLE AT THE LEG LEVEL

Here again, the distal hand grip, with the hand covering the heel and the forearm leaning on the plantar surface of the foot, allows you to resist both plantarflexion of the ankle and flexion of the knee. These two combined muscular actions put the investigated muscle under tension.

It is always helpful to alternate between movements of contraction and relaxation in order to perceive the muscular tension clearly.

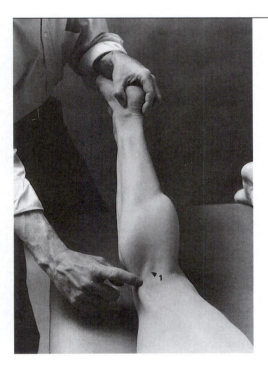

## FIGURE 10-28

### THE LATERAL HEAD OF THE GASTROCNEMIUS MUSCLE AT THE KNEE LEVEL AND THE POPLITEUS MUSCLE

The technique of placement under muscular tension is the same as that described above.

Like the medial head, the lateral head is attached, among other structures, to a reinforcement of the articular capsule on the posterior surface of the lateral condyle of the femur.

The proximal part of this muscle is a notable region in palpation anatomy, since it forms the inferolateral border of the popliteal fossa. This proximal muscular end is lined medially by the plantaris muscle (1), located in a deeper plane.

*Comment:*     *The muscular body of the popliteus muscle, located in the proximal and posterior portion of the leg, is approached indirectly through the muscular mass of the gastrocnemius muscle (palpation not demonstrated). Deep palpation of this region should be performed carefully in view of the presence of the tibial nerve. The tendon of this muscle is discussed in Fig. 7-25 in Part III, "The Knee."*

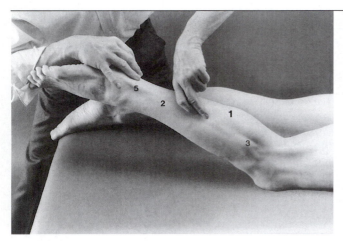

### FIGURE 10-29
### THE SOLEUS MUSCLE—THE PERONEAL HEAD IN ITS DISTAL PORTION (SEE COMMENT BELOW)

The distal end of the peroneal head of the soleus muscle is located above the peroneus brevis muscle (2) and behind the tendon of the peroneus longus muscle (3). Your distal hand covers the heel while your forearm is placed against the plantar surface of the foot to offer resistance to a plantarflexion. A contraction-relaxation sequence is ideal to perceive this muscular head well. It should be searched for along the fibula between the lateral head of the gastrocnemius muscle, located behind, and the peroneus longus muscle (3), located in front.

*Comment:* **The peroneal head of the soleus muscle is the part of the muscular body attaching to the fibula. It extends much more widely to the lateral surface of the leg than the tibial head to the medial aspect.**

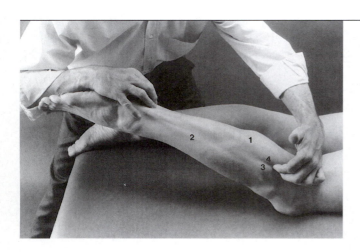

### FIGURE 10-30
### THE SOLEUS MUSCLE—THE PERONEAL HEAD IN ITS PROXIMAL PORTION (SEE COMMENT ABOVE)

The proximal and middle portions of the peroneal head of the soleus muscle (4) are located behind the peroneus longus muscle (3) and in front of the lateral head of the gastrocnemius muscle (1).

### FIGURES 10-29 AND 10-30

1. Lateral head of the gastrocnemius muscle
2. Peroneus brevis muscle
3. Peroneus longus muscle
4. Soleus muscle—peroneal head and tibial head
5. Tendon of the peroneus longus muscle
6. Medial head of the gastrocnemius muscle

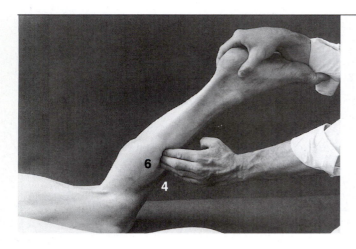

### FIGURE 10-31
### THE SOLEUS MUSCLE: THE TIBIAL HEAD

Your distal hand covers the calcaneum while your forearm is positioned against the plantar aspect of the foot in order to offer resistance to a plantarflexion of the ankle.

A contraction-relaxation sequence is ideal to perceive this muscular head well. It should be searched for along the medial border of the tibia up to its middle third, in front of the medial head of the gastrocnemius muscle (6).

*Comment:* **The tibial head (4), which is the portion of the muscular body attaching to the tibia, extends much less widely to the medial surface of the leg than the peroneal head to the lateral surface.**

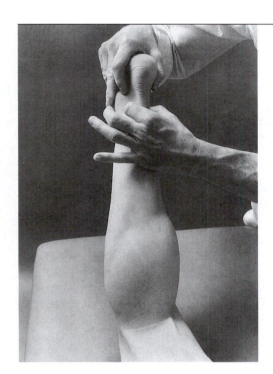

## FIGURE 10-32
### THE ACHILLES TENDON

The distal hand covers the heel and the forearm leans on the plantar surface of the foot, allowing the examiner to vary widely the degree of tension of the tendon.

The placement under tension may be done in two ways:

- by applying pressure on the plantar surface of the foot, bringing it in dorsiflexion and therefore stretching the tendon
- by using the technique of contraction-relaxation during plantarflexion of the foot

*Comment:*   *Once the tendon is located, the approach to it may also be carried out in the relaxed position and over its three surfaces (posterior, anterior, and lateral).*

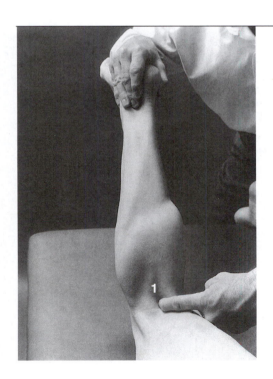

## FIGURE 10-33
### THE PLANTARIS MUSCLE IN THE POPLITEAL FOSSA

This muscle is located in front of the lateral head of the gastrocnemius muscle, beyond which it extends medially; it is not constant and is hardly accessible.

Your distal hand covers the heel while your forearm is applied against the plantar aspect of the foot, allowing a simultaneous resistance to plantarflexion of the foot and flexion of the knee.

The perception of the contraction of this muscle depends on the subject's morphology. The muscle (1) is perceived in the popliteal fossa, medial to the lateral head of the gastrocnemius muscle.

# DEEP PLANE

## THE POSTERIOR TIBIALIS MUSCLE

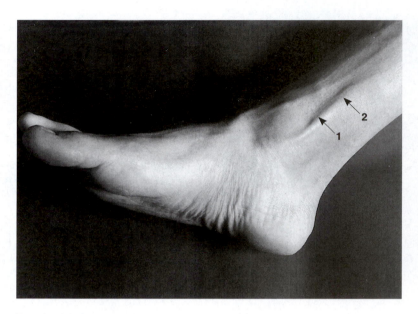

**FIGURE 10-34**
**MEDIAL VIEW OF THE INFERIOR THIRD OF THE LEG**

1. Tendon of the posterior tibialis muscle
2. Muscular body of the posterior tibialis muscle

*Comment:*     *Refer to page 124 to visualize the relations of this structure with the two other tendons of the medial retromalleolar groove, also belonging to the muscles of the deep plane of the leg:*

- *the flexor digitorum longus muscle*
- *the flexor hallucis longus muscle*

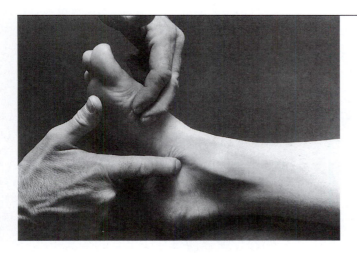

**FIGURE 10-35**

**THE TENDON OF THE POSTERIOR TIBIALIS MUSCLE BETWEEN THE TUBEROSITY OF THE NAVICULAR BONE AND THE MEDIAL MALLEOLUS**

Your distal hand guides and/or offers resistance to an adduction of the foot, positioned beforehand in plantarflexion. The tendon is perceived between the two structures mentioned above. It may be useful in certain cases to localize the tuberosity of the navicular bone. Consult Part V, "The Ankle and Foot."

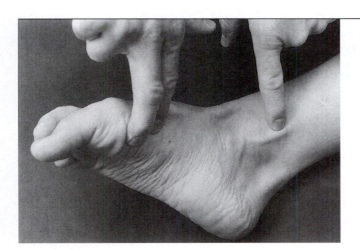

**FIGURE 10-36**

**THE TENDON OF THE POSTERIOR TIBIALIS MUSCLE AT THE ANKLE**

Your distal hand guides and/or offers resistance to adduction of the foot, positioned beforehand in plantarflexion. The tendon appears behind the medial malleolus. It is palpated as a very hard cylindrical cord.

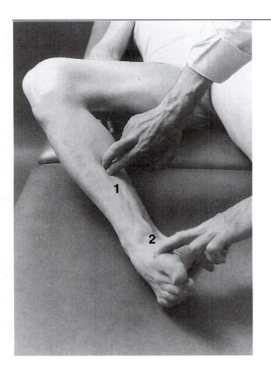

**FIGURE 10-37**

**THE TENDON AND THE MUSCULAR BODY OF THE POSTERIOR TIBIALIS MUSCLE IN THE LEG**

The subject's leg lies on its lateral aspect. To perceive the muscular contraction well, the digital grip is moved along the medial border of the tibia (1). The contraction is better perceived if a contraction-relaxation sequence is used. From an initial positioning of the foot in plantarflexion, the subject is asked to perform consecutive adductions against resistance. The muscular body that extends from the tendon (2) of the posterior tibialis muscle is situated in front of the flexor digitorum longus muscle up to the arch of the latter muscle, which is attached to the tibia at approximately 10 cm above the medial malleolus. After passing under this arch, the muscular body is located lateral to the flexor digitorum longus muscle. At this level, it is not directly approachable. It is covered by the triceps surae muscle.

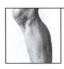

# THE FLEXOR DIGITORUM LONGUS MUSCLE

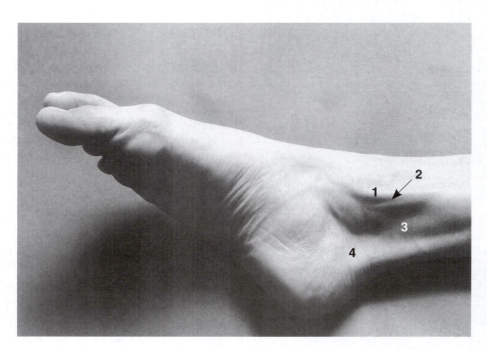

**FIGURE 10-38**
**MEDIAL VIEW OF THE LOWER THIRD OF THE LEG**

1.  Posterior tibialis muscle
2.  Flexor digitorum longus muscle
3.  Flexor hallucis longus muscle
4.  Achilles tendon

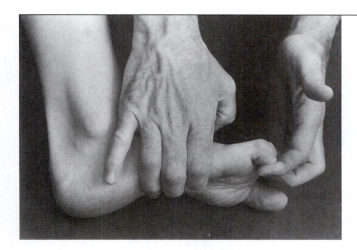

## FIGURE 10-39

### THE TENDONS OF THE FLEXOR DIGITORUM LONGUS MUSCLE AT THE LEVEL OF THE SOLE OF THE FOOT

Your distal hand guides and/or offers light resistance to alternate and rapid flexions of the toes, the ankle having been placed in neutral position earlier. The other hand is applied against the plantar aspect of the foot by covering its lateral border. The grip is wide in order to perceive the contraction well. The tendons themselves cannot be palpated directly, since they are covered by those of the flexor digitorum brevis muscle.

Comment:     *The muscular contraction involving these two muscles will be better perceived under the fingers if the proximal phalanges of the toes are positioned in hyperextension beforehand.*

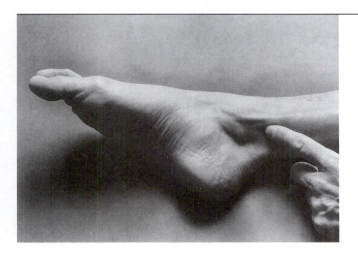

## FIGURE 10-40

### THE FLEXOR DIGITORUM LONGUS MUSCLE IN THE MEDIAL RETROMALLEOLAR GROOVE

The subject performs alternate and rapid flexions of the toes while the foot lies on the heel or on its lateral border.

The tendon is perceived in the area of the medial malleolus, behind the tendon of the posterior tibialis muscle.

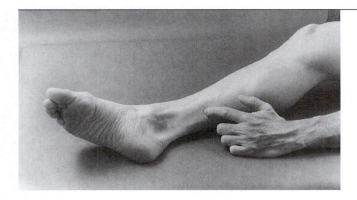

## FIGURE 10-41

### THE MUSCULAR BODY OF THE FLEXOR DIGITORUM LONGUS MUSCLE IN THE LOWER THIRD OF THE LEG

The leg lies on its lateral aspect and the ankle is in a relaxed position.

The index finger indicates the muscular body, which is located behind the posterior tibialis muscle up to an arch formed by the investigated muscle, which inserts into the tibia at approximately 10 cm above the medial malleolus. Above this arch, the muscular body is located medial to the posterior tibialis muscle.

The muscular contraction is better perceived if a sequence of contraction-relaxation is used. The subject is asked to perform rapidly consecutive flexions of the toes.

# THE FLEXOR HALLUCIS LONGUS MUSCLE

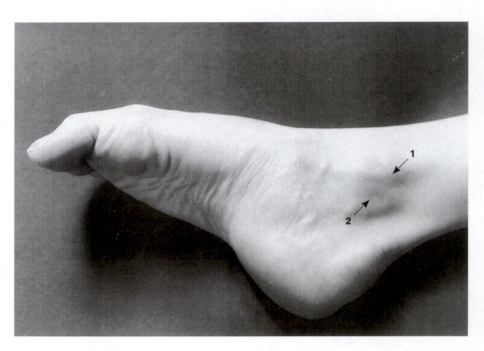

**FIGURE 10-42**
**MEDIAL VIEW OF THE LOWER THIRD OF THE LEG**

1. Tendon of the posterior tibialis muscle
2. Tendon of the flexor hallucis longus muscle

*Comment:* *Refer to page 124 to visualize the relations of this structure with the two other tendons of the medial retromalleolar groove also belonging to the muscles of the deep plane of the leg:*

- *the posterior tibialis muscle*
- *the flexor digitorum longus muscle*

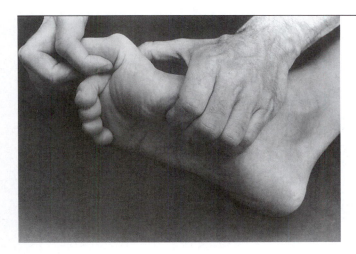

### FIGURE 10-43

### THE FLEXOR HALLUCIS LONGUS MUSCLE AT THE LEVEL OF THE SOLE OF THE FOOT

With the subject's ankle placed in neutral position and the foot lying on the heel or on its lateral border, your distal hand guides and/or offers light resistance to alternate and rapid flexions of the first toe. The other hand is positioned against the plantar aspect of the first metatarsal bone through a wide grip for a better perception of the contraction. This allows a better approach to the tendon, which is perceived somewhat as a cord beneath the fingers.

*Comment:*   *This tendinous structure will be perceived much better if the proximal phalanx of the first toe is placed in hyperextension beforehand.*

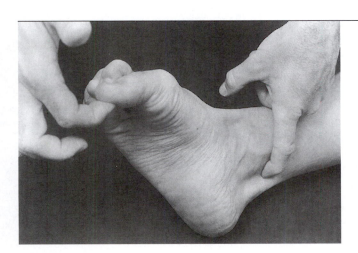

### FIGURE 10-44

### THE FLEXOR HALLUCIS LONGUS MUSCLE IN THE MEDIAL RETROMALLEOLAR GROOVE

Your distal hand guides and/or offers resistance to alternate and rapid flexions of the subject's first toe, the ankle having been placed in neutral position with the leg lying on its posterolateral surface. The muscle is palpated in the medial retromalleolar groove, between the medial malleolus and the Achilles tendon, and behind the tendon of the flexor digitorum longus muscle. See also Fig. 13-17 in Part V, "The Ankle and Foot," which follows.

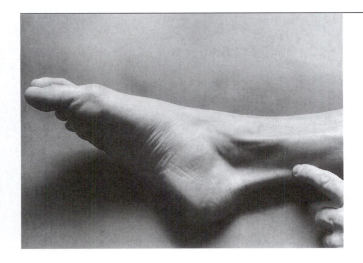

### FIGURE 10-45

### THE FLEXOR HALLUCIS LONGUS MUSCLE IN THE MEDIAL RETROMALLEOLAR GROOVE: VISUALIZATION OF THE MUSCULAR BODY

This figure simply allows a better visualization of the muscular body (indicated by the index finger), already investigated in Fig. 10-44 and located behind the flexor digitorum longus muscle (2) (see Fig. 10-38).

The contraction is better perceived if the subject is asked to perform consecutive flexions of the first toe.

# THE ANKLE AND FOOT

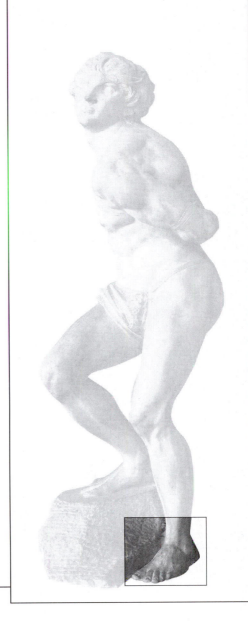

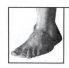
## ILLUSTRATED STUDY OF THE ANKLE/FOOT (ANTERIOR)

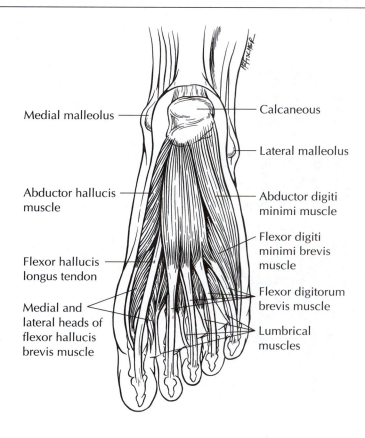

Medial malleolus

Calcaneous

Lateral malleolus

Abductor hallucis muscle

Abductor digiti minimi muscle

Flexor digiti minimi brevis muscle

Flexor hallucis longus tendon

Flexor digitorum brevis muscle

Medial and lateral heads of flexor hallucis brevis muscle

Lumbrical muscles

## ILLUSTRATED STUDY OF THE ANKLE/FOOT (DORSUM)

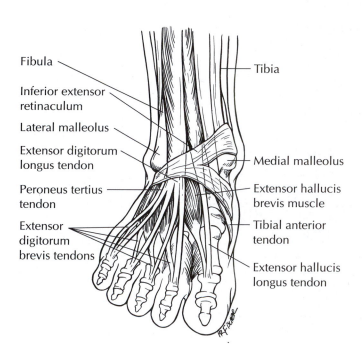

Fibula

Tibia

Inferior extensor retinaculum

Lateral malleolus

Extensor digitorum longus tendon

Medial malleolus

Peroneus tertius tendon

Extensor hallucis brevis muscle

Extensor digitorum brevis tendons

Tibial anterior tendon

Extensor hallucis longus tendon

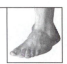

## ILLUSTRATED STUDY OF THE ANKLE/FOOT (LATERAL)

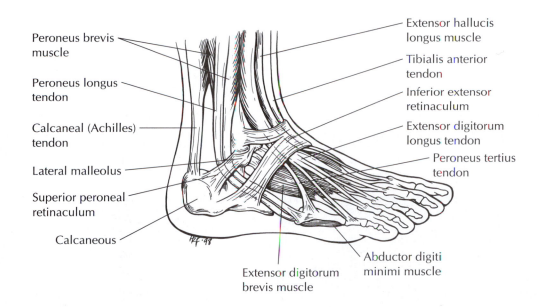

Peroneus brevis muscle

Peroneus longus tendon

Calcaneal (Achilles) tendon

Lateral malleolus

Superior peroneal retinaculum

Calcaneous

Extensor hallucis longus muscle

Tibialis anterior tendon

Inferior extensor retinaculum

Extensor digitorum longus tendon

Peroneus tertius tendon

Extensor digitorum brevis muscle

Abductor digiti minimi muscle

## ILLUSTRATED STUDY OF THE ANKLE/FOOT (MEDIAL)

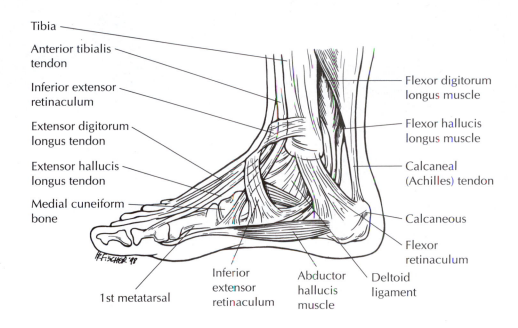

Tibia

Anterior tibialis tendon

Inferior extensor retinaculum

Extensor digitorum longus tendon

Extensor hallucis longus tendon

Medial cuneiform bone

Flexor digitorum longus muscle

Flexor hallucis longus muscle

Calcaneal (Achilles) tendon

Calcaneous

Flexor retinaculum

1st metatarsal

Inferior extensor retinaculum

Abductor hallucis muscle

Deltoid ligament

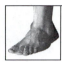

# TOPOGRAPHIC PRESENTATION OF THE FOOT

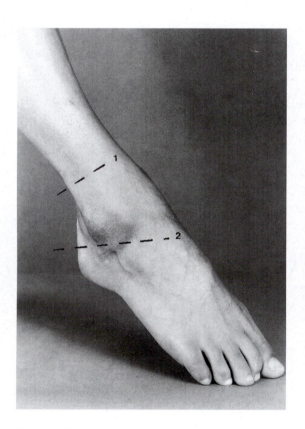

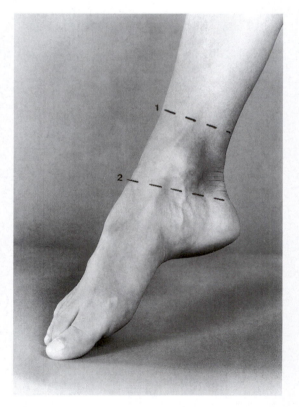

**FIGURE 11-1**
**ANTEROLATERAL VIEW OF THE ANKLE AND OF THE FOOT**

1. Superior border of the region of the ankle

**FIGURE 11-2**
**ANTEROMEDIAL VIEW OF THE ANKLE AND OF THE FOOT**

2. Inferior border of the region of the ankle

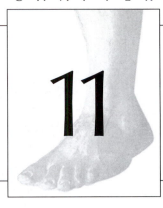

# 11

# OSTEOLOGY

## THE LATERAL BORDER

The bony structures accessible by palpation are as follows:

- The fifth metatarsal bone:
  —the head (Fig. 11-4)
  —the lateral surface of the shaft (Fig. 11-5)
  —the inferior border of the shaft (Fig. 11-6)
  —the base of the fifth metatarsal bone: located by a global approach to the lateral border of the foot (Fig. 11-7)
  —the styloid process or tubercular eminence of the fifth metatarsal bone (Fig. 11-8)

- The cuboid bone:
  —the lateral border (Fig. 11-9; also see Fig. 11-7)
  —the dorsal surface (Fig. 11-10)
  —the plantar surface (Fig. 11-11)

- The calcaneus:
  —the lateral surface (Fig. 11-12)
  —the greater process (Fig. 11-13; also see Fig. 11-7)
  —the cuboid facet or the anterior surface (Fig. 11-14)

  —the floor of the sinus tarsi (Fig. 11-15)
  —the peroneal tubercle (Fig. 11-16)
  —the tubercle of insertion of the calcaneofibular ligament (Fig. 11-17)
  —the posterior portion of the lateral surface (Fig. 11-18)
  —the superior surface: the lateral portion of the posterior segment (Fig. 11-19)

- The talus:
  —the lateral surface of the neck (Fig. 11-20; also see Fig. 11-7)
  —the lateral process (Fig. 11-21)

- The lateral malleolus:
  —the anterior border (Fig. 11-22)
  —the apex (Fig. 11-23)
  —the posterior border (Fig. 11-24).

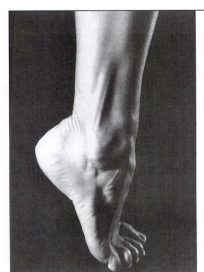

**FIGURE 11-3**
**THE LATERAL SURFACE OF THE ANKLE AND OF THE FOOT**

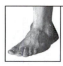

# THE FIFTH METATARSAL BONE

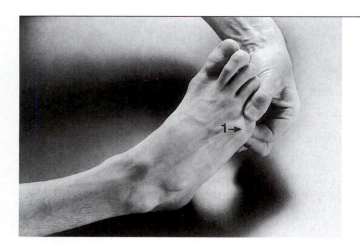

## FIGURE 11-4
### THE HEAD OF THE FIFTH METATARSAL BONE

The fifth toe should be brought into plantarflexion in order to demonstrate the head (1) of the fifth metatarsal bone on the dorsal portion of the lateral border of the foot. This demonstration also allows the localization of the metatarsophalangeal joint.

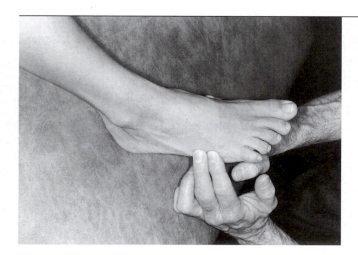

## FIGURE 11-5
### THE LATERAL SURFACE OF THE SHAFT OF THE FIFTH METATARSAL BONE

Directly under the skin, there is no difficulty in following it since it is located just above the abductor muscle of the fifth toe (abductor digiti minimi).

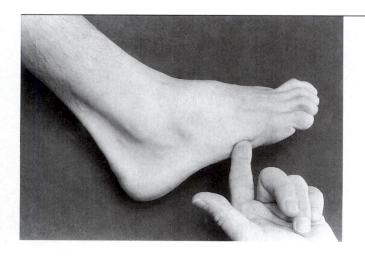

## FIGURE 11-6
### THE INFERIOR BORDER OF THE SHAFT OF THE FIFTH METATARSAL BONE

The inferior border of the shaft is palpated by the index finger as a slightly curved structure with a plantar concavity, which is well perceived. In this picture, the index finger pushes away the abductor muscle of the fifth toe in order to be in contact with the investigated bony structure.

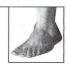

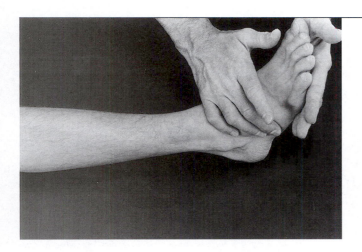

## FIGURE 11-7

**THE BASE OF THE FIFTH METATARSAL BONE, LOCALIZED BY A GLOBAL APPROACH TO THE LATERAL BORDER OF THE FOOT**

The foot is in a relaxed position, lying on a table or on your knee. Your proximal hand is placed on the proximal aspect of the foot, gently covering the lateral border of the foot. The lateral border of the little finger is placed against the lateral malleolus.

In this case, the little finger is in contact with the greater process of the calcaneus. The ring finger faces the cuboid bone. The middle finger faces the base of the fifth metatarsal bone.

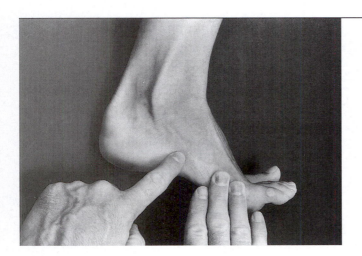

## FIGURE 11-8

**TUBEROSITY OF THE FIFTH METATARSAL BONE**

Articulating its posterior extremity with the cuboid bone, the fifth metatarsal bone has the peculiarity of presenting a prominent process behind, below, and outside its base. It is into this tubercular eminence that the tendon of the peroneus brevis muscle is inserted. Posteriorly, this process partially overlooks the lateral border of the cuboid bone.

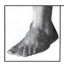
# THE CUBOID BONE

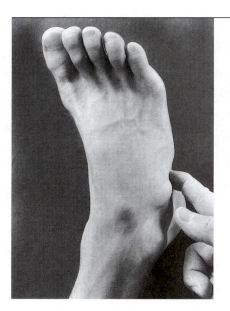

### FIGURE 11-9
#### THE LATERAL BORDER OF THE CUBOID BONE (SEE FIG. 11-7)

In the posterior aspect of the foot the cuboid bone is the bony structure immediately following the styloid process of the fifth metatarsal bone (Figs. 11-7 and 11-8). Once this process is located, your fingers should slide posteriorly into a depression over the lateral border of the foot, to be in contact with a ridge that represents the investigated structure.

*Comment:* *The tendon of the peroneus brevis muscle, which runs along this ridge, hampers the investigation unless it is relaxed.*

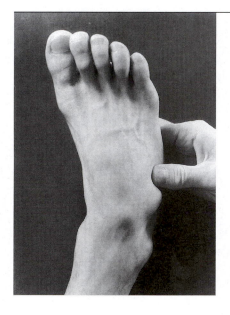

### FIGURE 11-10
#### THE DORSAL SURFACE OF THE CUBOID BONE

The two bony structures used for proper positioning on this surface are:

- the tuberosity of the fifth metatarsal bone, already located (Figs. 11-7 and 11-8),
- the greater process of the calcaneus (Fig. 11-13). The dorsal surface of the cuboid bone is obviously located between these two structures, which represent its anterior and posterior borders.

Your thumb should first be placed on the lateral border of the cuboid bone (Fig. 11-9), then moved slightly toward the dorsal surface of the foot in order to be in contact with the investigated bony structure.

*Comment:* *Rough, directed downward and laterally, it is directly under the skin and easy to palpate. The tendon of the peroneus brevis muscle runs along its lateral aspect and the extensor digitorum brevis muscle partially covers it.*

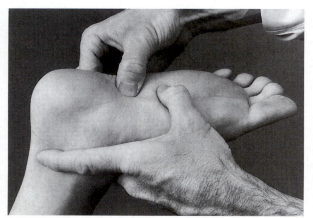

### FIGURE 11-11
#### THE PLANTAR SURFACE OF THE CUBOID BONE

After localizing the styloid process or tubercular eminence of the fifth metatarsal bone (Figs. 11-7 and 11-8) and the greater process of the calcaneus (Figs. 11-7 and 11-13), your thumb is placed between the two structures, and then moved around the lateral border of the foot and the lateral border of the cuboid bone to be positioned on the plantar surface of this bone.

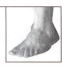

# THE CALCANEUS

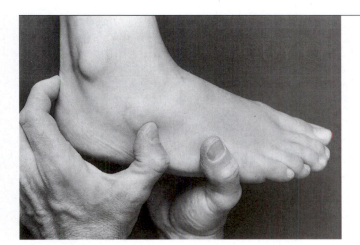

### FIGURE 11-12
### THE LATERAL SURFACE OF THE CALCANEUS

The forefoot is adducted and supinated in order to project the anterior articular surface of the calcaneus and to partially uncover it.

Your thumb is positioned on this surface and the index finger on the posterior surface of the calcaneus in order to clearly perceive the dimension of this bone among the bones of the foot.

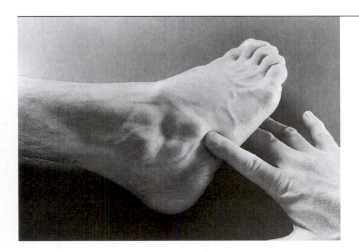

### FIGURE 11-13
### THE GREATER PROCESS OF THE CALCANEUS (SEE ALSO FIG. 11-7)

It delimits the lateral calcaneocuboidal interspace posteriorly. A supination of the forefoot facilitates its access. It may be very prominent in certain subjects, as is the case in this figure.

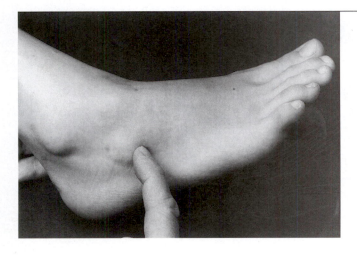

### FIGURE 11-14
### THE ANTERIOR (ARTICULAR) SURFACE OR CUBOID FACET OF THE CALCANEUS

In order to uncover the superior anterolateral portion of this facet, it is usually sufficient to ask the subject to adduct and supinate the forefoot placed in slight flexion.

If this is not sufficient, it is possible to perform this maneuver using a passive technique. One hand is used to stabilize the calcaneus while the other hand brings the forefoot into adduction, supination, and slight plantarflexion (also see Fig. 11-7).

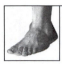

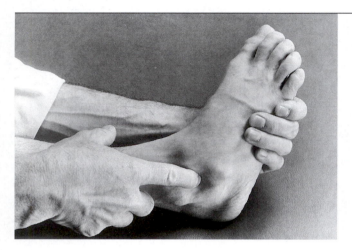

## Figure 11-15
### The floor of the sinus tarsi

Anatomic reminder: The sinus tarsi is formed by the interlocking of the calcaneus and of the talus. It becomes progressively wider as it runs outward and forward. Its floor is the calcaneal sulcus, while its roof is the sulcus tali. The superposition of these two grooves forms a conduit called the sinus tarsi. The sinus itself is therefore not accessible, but its floor is, exactly where it opens on the superior surface of the calcaneus at the level of its anterior segment.

*Comment:* *The posterior portion of the sinus tarsi is occupied by the two or three bundles of the calcaneotalar ligament.*

Technique of approach: With the subject's foot in neutral position, place your index finger on the anterior border of the lateral malleolus. As the finger is advanced slightly toward the sole of the foot, the investigated structure is palpated as a depression. The extensor digitorum brevis muscle may hamper this approach (one should make sure it is relaxed). The tendon of the extensor digitorum longus muscle as well as the lateral aspect of the neck of the talus are located medially.

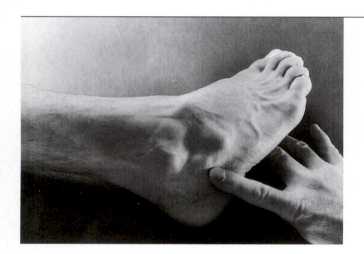

## Figure 11-16
### The peroneal trochlea

This is a bony prominence located approximately one fingerbreadth below the lateral malleolus. The peroneal trochlea separates the underlying groove of the peroneus longus muscle from the overlying groove of the peroneus brevis muscle. It is palpated approximately one fingerbreadth from the apex of the lateral malleolus (also see Figs. 11-12 and 11-23).

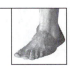

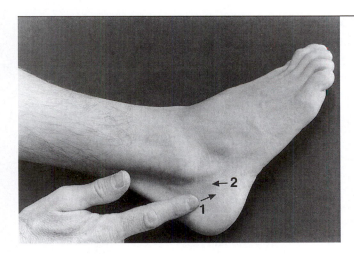

### Figure 11-17
### Tubercle of insertion of the calcaneofibular ligament

This structure is not always well differentiated. It is the site of insertion for the middle fasciculus or calcaneofibular ligament of the lateral lateral ligament of the ankle. With the subject's foot in neutral position (0°), the tubercle is located behind the peroneal tubercle (2) (Fig. 11-16) at approximately one fingerbreadth below and one fingerbreadth behind the lateral calcaneotalar articular interspace.

*Comment:* ***The tubercle is not constant. In its absence, the calcaneofibular ligament inserts directly into the lateral surface of the calcaneus.***

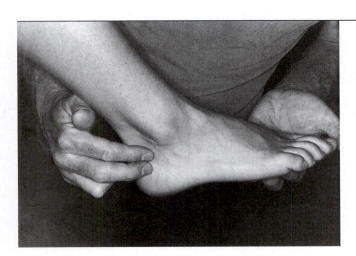

### Figure 11-18
### The posterior portion of the lateral surface of the calcaneus

This structure is perceived beneath the fingers as flat and rough over essentially the entire lateral surface of the calcaneus, which is directly under the skin. In this figure, the grip is somewhat withdrawn in order to demonstrate as widely as possible the bony structure discussed.

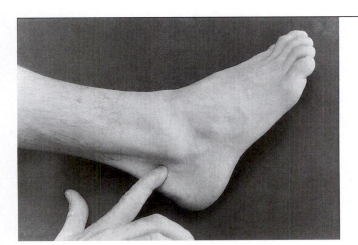

### Figure 11-19
### The lateral portion of the posterior segment of the calcaneus—posterior surface

In this figure, the index finger lies on the bony structure mentioned above (Fig. 11-18), behind the talus and lateral to the Achilles tendon.

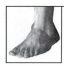 

# THE TALUS

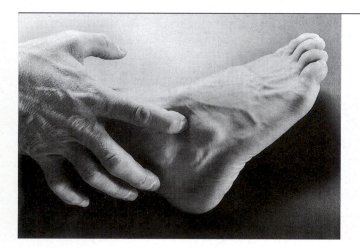

### FIGURE 11-20
### THE LATERAL SURFACE OF THE NECK OF THE TALUS (SEE ALSO FIG. 11-7)

The subject's foot is first placed in neutral position. Your index finger is placed on the anterior border of the lateral malleolus. On being advanced slightly forward and inward, it faces the investigated structure. Tip the forefoot over in slight supination to make the lateral surface more accessible.

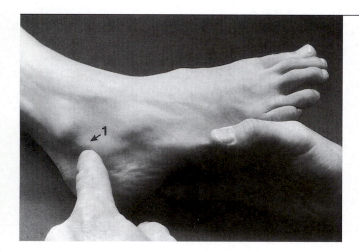

### FIGURE 11-21
### THE LATERAL PROCESS OF THE TALUS

This structure is a tubercle located in front of the peroneal tubercle and under the lateral calcaneotalar interspace. With the subject's foot in neutral position (0°), apply your index finger against the posterior portion of the inferior or distal end of the fibula. This tubercle is palpated approximately one fingerbreadth in front of the peroneal tubercle.

*Comment:*    *In this figure, the index finger is displaced backward, in order not to hamper visualization of the investigated structure (1).*

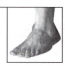

# THE LATERAL MALLEOLUS

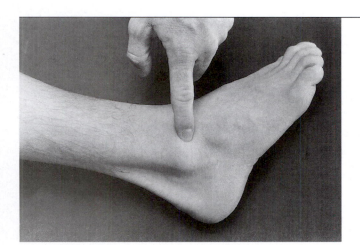

### FIGURE 11-22
#### THE ANTERIOR BORDER OF THE LATERAL MALLEOLUS

In its uppermost portion, this is the site of insertion of the anterior tibiofibular ligament. In its lowermost or distal portion, it is the site of insertion of the anterior talofibular fibular ligament and of the calcaneofibular ligament.

*Comment:* *These last two ligaments are respectively the anterior and middle fasciculi of the lateral lateral ligament.*

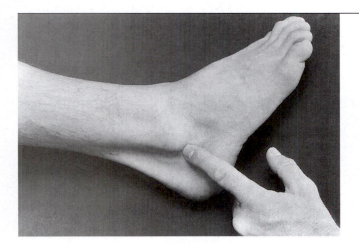

### FIGURE 11-23
#### THE APEX OF THE LATERAL MALLEOLUS

The apex presents, just in front of its most prominent point, a groove for the attachment of a part of the middle fasciculus (calcaneofibular ligament) of the lateral lateral ligament of the ankle. The other portion of this ligament is located on the lowermost portion of the apex's anterior border.

It is therefore an important landmark for localizing the fibular insertions of this ligament.

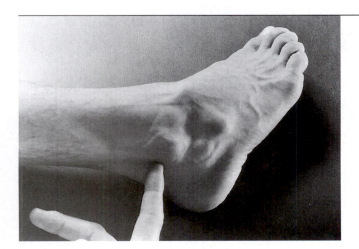

### FIGURE 11-24
#### THE POSTERIOR BORDER OF THE LATERAL MALLEOLUS

One must ensure that the peroneus muscles (peroneus longus and peroneus brevis) are relaxed to prevent their tendons, passing behind this border, from hampering its access.

*Comment:* *This border is the site of attachment of the posterior tibiofibular ligament as well as the posterior fasciculus (posterior talofibular-fibular ligament) of the lateral lateral ligament of the ankle.*

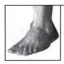

# THE MEDIAL BORDER

The bony structures accessible by palpation are as follows:

- The first metatarsal bone
  —the phalanges of the first toe and the head of the metatarsal bone: dorsal approach (Fig. 11-26)
  —the head of the metatarsal bone: plantar approach (Fig. 11-27)
  —the shaft (Figs. 11-28 through 11-31)
  —the base: located by a global approach to the medial border of the foot (Fig. 11-32)
  —the posteromedial tubercle (Fig. 11-33)
  —the posterolateral tubercle (Fig. 11-34)

- The medial cuneiform bone
  —the medial surface, located by using the anterior tibialis muscle (Fig. 11-35; also see Fig. 11-32)
  —the superior surface (Fig. 11-36)

- The navicular bone
  —the tuberosity of the navicular bone: direct approach (Fig. 11-37; see also Fig. 11-32)

—the tuberosity of the navicular bone, located by using the posterior tibialis muscle (Fig. 11-38)

- The talus
  —the ligamentous field or middle field of the head of the talus (Fig. 11-39; see also Fig. 11-32)
  —the neck of the talus (Figs. 11-40 and 11-41; see also Fig. 11-32)
  —the posteromedial tubercle (Fig. 11-42)
  —the posterolateral tubercle (Fig. 11-43)

- The calcaneus
  —the lesser process (Fig. 11-44)
  —the groove of the calcaneus (Fig. 11-45)

- The medial malleolus
  —the anterior border (Fig. 11-46)
  —the inferior extremity (Fig. 11-47)
  —the posterior border (Fig. 11-48)

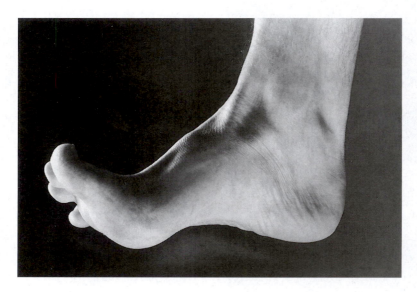

**FIGURE 11-25**
**THE MEDIAL BORDER OF THE FOOT**

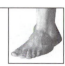

# THE FIRST METATARSAL BONE

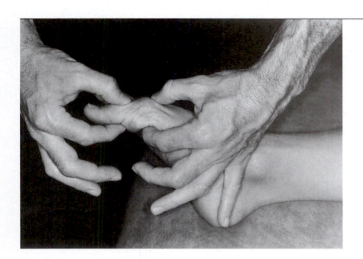

### FIGURE 11-26

### THE PHALANGES OF THE FIRST TOE AND THE HEAD OF THE FIRST METATARSAL BONE—DORSAL APPROACH

The phalanges are not difficult to examine. Remember that each toe except for the first is composed of three phalanges, while the first toe has two.

A precise palpation allows the examiner to perceive the medial and lateral surfaces as well as the plantar and dorsal surfaces of the shaft of each phalanx of the first toe.

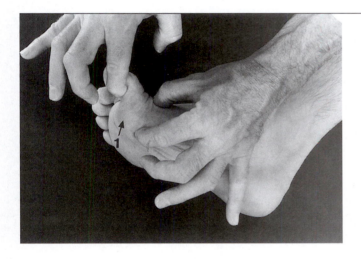

### FIGURE 11-27

### THE HEAD AND THE SESAMOID BONES OF THE FIRST METATARSAL BONE—PLANTAR APPROACH

Placing your distal digital grip on the plantar aspect of the proximal phalanx, bring it into extension. You will then palpate the plantar base of this phalanx—the inferior or plantar articular surface of the head of the first metatarsal bone and the two sesamoid bones.

Comment:     *The anterior extremity or head of each metatarsal bone ends by a convex articular surface, which is much larger in its plantar (1) than its dorsal portion. This grip allows you to free up the articular surface.*

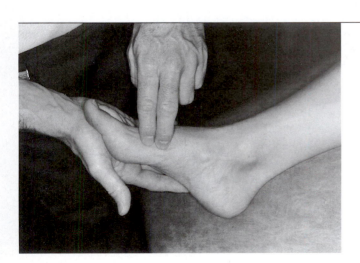

### FIGURE 11-28

### THE MEDIAL BORDER OF THE FIRST METATARSAL BONE

This border is located over the medial aspect of the foot. Directly under the skin, it has the characteristic of being situated in the dorsal half of the medial border of the foot.

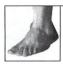

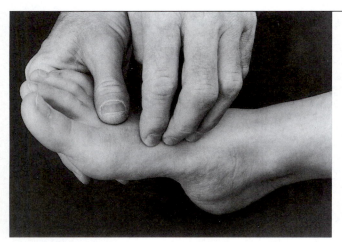

### FIGURE 11-29
#### THE DORSAL SURFACE OF THE FIRST METATARSAL BONE

The shaft of each metatarsal bone is prismoid and triangular in shape. This shaft presents a dorsal surface that is generally narrow but much wider in the back than in the front.

*Comment:*     *An anatomic characteristic of all metatarsal bones is the presence of two borders for each dorsal surface, medial and lateral.*

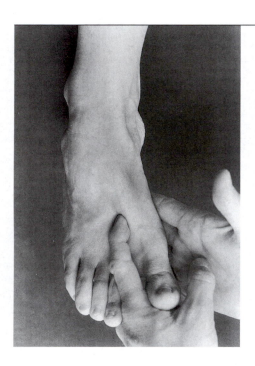

### FIGURE 11-30
#### THE LATERAL SURFACE OF THE FIRST METATARSAL BONE

The lateral facet of each metatarsal bone demarcates respectively with the medial facet of the adjacent metatarsal bone a particular space called the interosseus or metatarsal interspace.

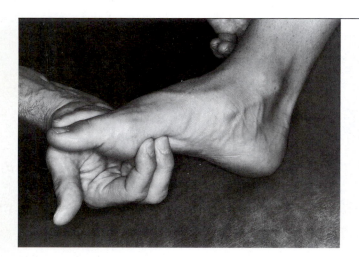

### FIGURE 11-31
#### THE INFERIOR BORDER OF THE SHAFT OF THE FIRST METATARSAL BONE

The inferior or plantar border of the shaft of the first metatarsal bone is clearly palpated as a curved structure with plantar concavity (Figs. 11-4 and 11-7).

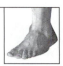

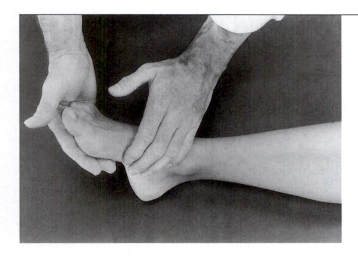

## FIGURE 11-32

### THE BASE OF THE FIRST METATARSAL BONE—LOCATED THROUGH A GLOBAL APPROACH TO THE MEDIAL BORDER OF THE FOOT

The subject's foot is in a normal, relaxed position, lying on a table or on the knee of the examiner.

Your proximal hand is positioned on the proximal aspect of the foot and gently covers its medial border. The ulnar side of the small finger is placed on the anterior border of the medial malleolus.

In this case:

- the small finger faces the medial surface of the neck of the talus
- the ring finger faces the navicular bone
- the middle finger faces the medial cuneiform bone
- the index finger faces the base of the first metatarsal bone

*Comment:*    *This global approach of the bony structures of the medial border of the foot may be considered to be reliable in most subjects.*

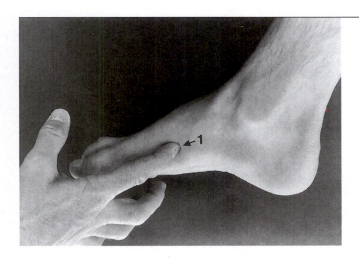

## FIGURE 11-33

### THE POSTEROMEDIAL TUBERCLE OF THE BASE OF THE FIRST METATARSAL BONE

The metatarsal extension of the anterior tibialis muscle inserts into this tubercle. Its other site of distal insertion is the inferior portion of the medial cuneiform bone (1) (Fig. 11-35).

Your index finger slides between the muscular body of the abductor hallucis muscle and the plantar border of the first metatarsal bone, which is palpated as a curved structure (Fig. 11-31). This tubercle may be found near the base of the metatarsal bone by following the medial border of its shaft.

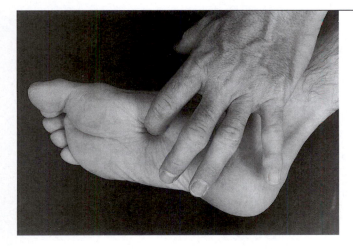

## FIGURE 11-34

### THE POSTEROLATERAL TUBERCLE OF THE FIRST METATARSAL BONE

Located below, outside, and behind the previous tubercle, this tubercle receives the main distal extension of the peroneus longus muscle.

It is obvious that this bony prominence, covered by the soft tissues, will be better perceived in a case of muscular wasting, which occurs when a person is bedridden for a long period. In the opposite case, the pressure applied must be quite firm in order to perceive the investigated structure.

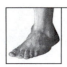

# THE MEDIAL CUNEIFORM BONE

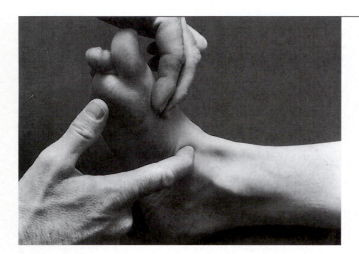

**FIGURE 11-35**

**THE MEDIAL CUNEIFORM BONE: THE MEDIAL SURFACE**
**(SEE ALSO FIG. 11-32)**

An effective technique to localize this surface is to place the anterior tibialis muscle under tension, asking the subject to perform a supination and dorsiflexion of the foot with or without resistance. The investigated surface is then easy to locate, since this muscle attaches to its anteroinferior portion.

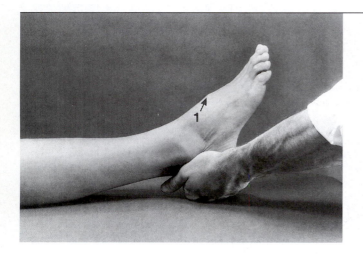

**FIGURE 11-36**

**LATERAL VIEW OF THE SUPERIOR BORDER OF THE MEDIAL CUNEIFORM BONE**

Positioned on the medial border of the foot, between the navicular bone and the first metatarsal bone, the medial cuneiform bone presents a sharp superior or dorsal border (1) resembling a fish bone, particularly in its posterior aspect.

*Comment:*     ***This characteristic is demonstrated in this picture by a lateral view.***

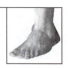

# THE NAVICULAR BONE

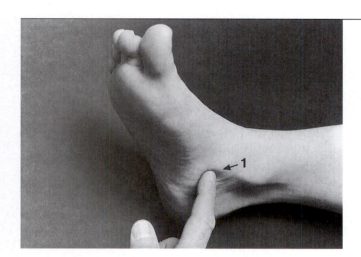

### FIGURE 11-37

### THE TUBEROSITY OF THE NAVICULAR BONE—DIRECT APPROACH (SEE ALSO FIG. 11-32)

This tuberosity projects over the inferior portion of the medial surface of the navicular bone (1). It is the site of insertion of the posterior tibialis muscle.

It is accessible just behind and medial to the tendon of the anterior tibialis muscle (see Fig 11-59). In many subjects, this tuberosity is clearly visible, as in this picture.

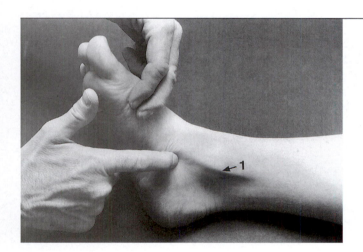

### FIGURE 11-38

### THE TUBEROSITY OF THE NAVICULAR BONE: LOCALIZATION BY USING THE POSTERIOR TIBIALIS MUSCLE

Placing the posterior tibialis muscle (1) under tension is an effective method of locating the tuberosity of the navicular bone when it is less apparent.

The foot is positioned in plantarflexion beforehand and the subject is asked to perform an adduction of the foot.

From the medial malleolus, follow the tendon of the muscle mentioned above downward to the investigated tuberosity.

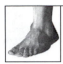

# THE TALUS

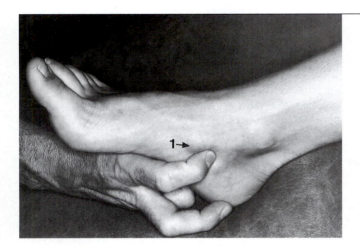

### FIGURE 11-39

### THE LIGAMENTOUS FIELD OR MIDDLE FIELD OF THE HEAD OF THE TALUS (SEE ALSO FIG. 11-32)

As indicated by its name, this structure is in relation with the inferior or plantar calcaneonavicular ligament.

It is located behind the anterosuperior field of the head of the talus, which articulates with the navicular bone.

Position your finger behind the tuberosity of the navicular bone (1), over the medial border of the foot, to perceive this smooth surface under the finger.

Comment: *Depending on the subject, it is sometimes useful to abduct and pronate the forefoot in order to better palpate this structure.*

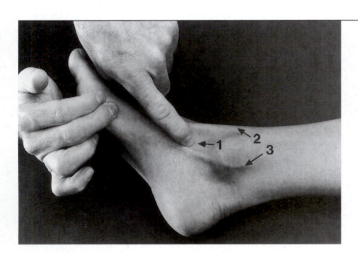

### FIGURE 11-40

### THE MEDIAL PORTION OF THE NECK OF THE TALUS (SEE ALSO FIG. 11-32)

The medial aspect of the neck of the talus (1) is essentially examined between the tendons of the anterior tibialis muscle (2) laterally and of the posterior tibialis muscle (3) medially.

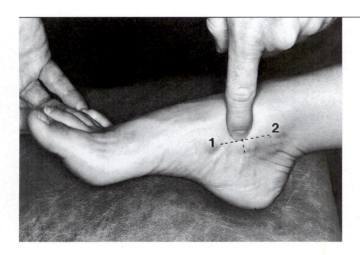

### FIGURE 11-41

### THE MEDIAL PORTION OF THE NECK OF THE TALUS (SECOND METHOD)

In addition to a localization by using the tendons (figure above), it is also possible to locate this structure through an imaginary line drawn between the tuberosity of the navicular bone (1) and the medial malleolus (2).

From the middle of this line and toward the malleolus (2), you face the neck of the talus (rough surface under the fingers).

From the middle of this line and toward the tuberosity of the navicular bone (1), one faces the ligamentous field of the head of the talus (structure perceived as smooth under the fingers) (Fig. 11-39).

Comment: *A rough ridge, more or less prominent depending on the subject, separates these two portions of the talus: the head and the neck.*

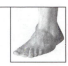

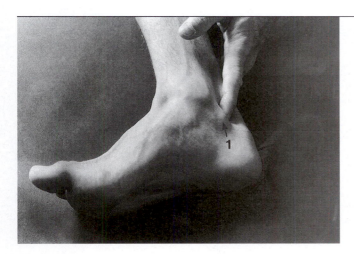

### Figure 11-42
#### The medial tubercle of the talus

It is important to remember that this bony structure (1) belongs to the posterior surface of the talus and that it is the site of insertion of the posterior talofibular fasciculus, the deep layer of the deltoid ligament.

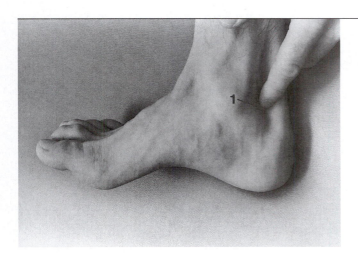

### Figure 11-43
#### The lateral tubercle of the talus

This tubercle (1) also belongs to the posterior surface of the talus. Your finger should be placed against the Achilles tendon, and, to investigate, the posterior border of the talus should be approached.

*Comment:*     *In most subjects, this structure is difficult to access, but it is a remarkable bony structure, since it is the site of insertion of the posterior talofibular-fibular ligament, posterior fasciculus of the lateral lateral ligament of the ankle.*

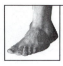
# THE CALCANEUS

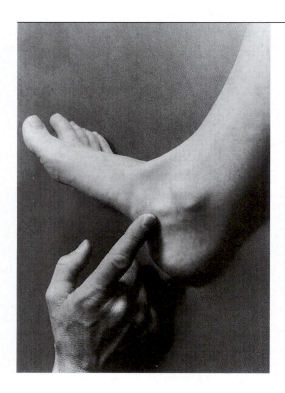

### FIGURE 11-44
#### SUSTENTACULUM TALI

This structure is located approximately one fingerbreadth below the medial malleolus. Its superior portion supports the medial articular surface of the calcaneus, intended for the talus.

When this process is approached, the medial calcaneotalar interspace is very close.

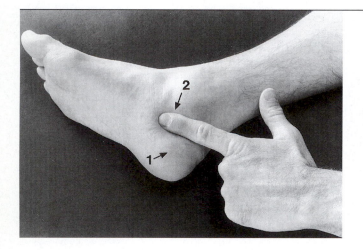

### FIGURE 11-45
#### THE GROOVE OF THE CALCANEUS

Directed downward and forward, it occupies the width of the medial surface. It is limited posteriorly and inferiorly by the posteromedial tuberosity of the calcaneus (1) and anteriorly and superiorly by a projection, the size of which depends on the subject: sustentaculum tali (2).

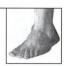

# THE MEDIAL MALLEOLUS

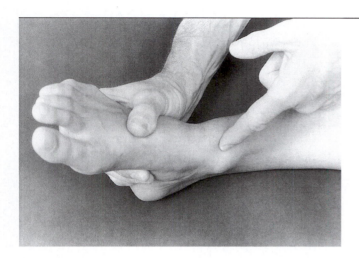

### FIGURE 11-46
### THE ANTERIOR BORDER OF THE MEDIAL MALLEOLUS

Very thick and rough, this is the site of insertion of the superficial layer of the medial lateral ligament of the ankle.

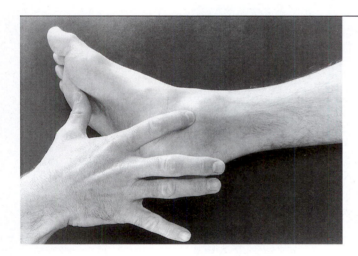

### FIGURE 11-47
### THE INFERIOR EXTREMITY OF THE MEDIAL MALLEOLUS

This structure is formed by two tubercles (anterior and posterior) separated by a depression, which is the site of insertion of the superficial and deep layers of the medial lateral ligament of the ankle.

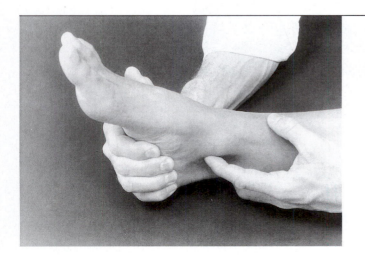

### FIGURE 11-48
### THE POSTERIOR BORDER OF THE MEDIAL MALLEOLUS

This structure presents a malleolar sulcus directed downward and medially. It is accessible for examination if the tendons contained in it are maintained in a relaxed position. The tendon of the posterior tibialis muscle is the most anterior and that of the flexor digitorum longus muscle the most posterior.

*Comment:* **In fact, these two tendons travel behind the medial malleolus in their respective osteofibrous sheaths.**

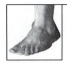

# THE ANTERIOR SURFACE OF THE ANKLE AND THE DORSAL SURFACE OF THE FOOT

The structures accessible by palpation are as follows:

- the heads of the metatarsal bones in dorsal view (Fig. 11-50)
- the fifth metatarsal bone (Fig. 11-51)
- the fourth metatarsal bone (Fig. 11-52)
- the third metatarsal bone (Fig. 11-53)

- the second metatarsal bone (Fig. 11-54)
- the first metatarsal bone (Fig. 11-55)
- the neck of the talus (Fig. 11-56)
- the anterior border of the lower extremity of the tibia (Fig. 11-57)

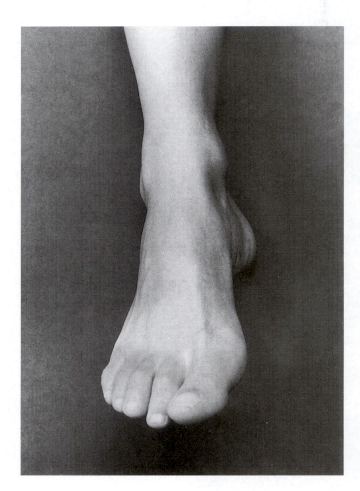

**FIGURE 11-49**
**ANTERIOR VIEW OF THE ANKLE AND DORSAL VIEW OF THE FOOT**

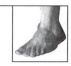

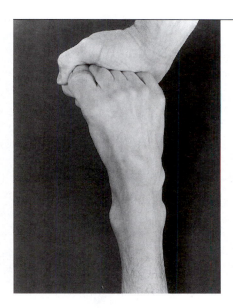

## FIGURE 11-50
### THE HEADS OF THE METATARSAL BONES—DORSAL VIEW

By taking a global grip of all toes, carry out a plantarflexion that will be sufficient to project the metatarsal heads. This maneuver can obviously be performed for each metatarsal bone separately.

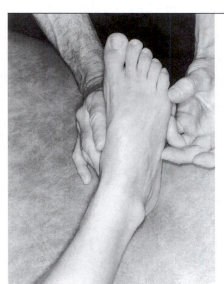

## FIGURE 11-51
### THE FIFTH METATARSAL BONE

First the head (see Fig. 11-4) is located as well as the base (see Figs. 11-7 and 11-8). After positioning the head on the related articular interspace (Fig. 12-7), the fifth metatarsal bone may be grabbed between the thumb and the index finger.

It is interesting to note the position and the dimension of this bone relative to the other metatarsal bones. It faces the cuboid bone posteriorly and the fourth metatarsal bone medially. Its posterolateral aspect shows a styloid process also called the tuberosity of the fifth metatarsal bone.

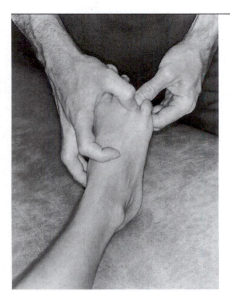

## FIGURE 11-52
### THE FOURTH METATARSAL BONE

The head and the base are located after locating the related articular interspace (Fig. 12-8).

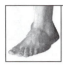

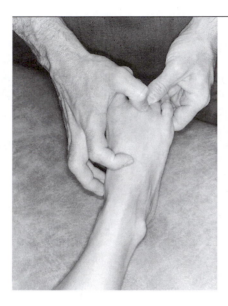

## FIGURE 11-53
### THE THIRD METATARSAL BONE

The head and the base are located after locating the related articular interspace (Fig. 12-9).

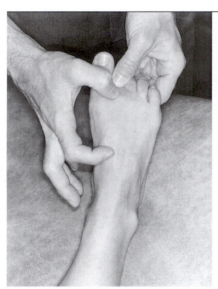

## FIGURE 11-54
### THE SECOND METATARSAL BONE

The head and the base are located after locating the related articular interspace (Fig. 12-10).

*Comment:*     *This is the longest of the metatarsal bones.*

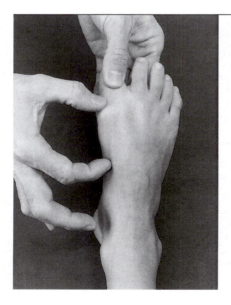

## FIGURE 11-55
### THE FIRST METATARSAL BONE

The head (Fig. 11-26) and the base (Figs. 11-32 and 11-33) are located after locating the related articular interspace (Figs. 11-32 and 12-11).

*Comment:*     *This is the shortest and the broadest of the metatarsal bones.*

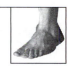

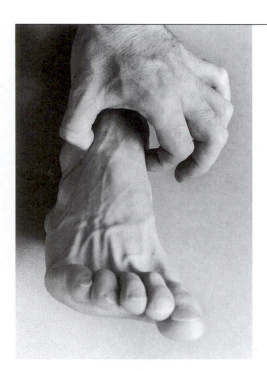

### FIGURE 11-56
### THE NECK OF THE TALUS

In this picture, the neck of the talus is grabbed through its medial and lateral surfaces. The thumb is positioned on the lateral surface and the index finger on the medial surface [these two portions of the neck were seen during the examination of the lateral (Figs. 11-7 and 11-20) and medial (Figs. 11-32, 11-40, and 11-41) borders of the foot, respectively].

The superior surface of the neck of the talus is located between the thumb and the index finger.

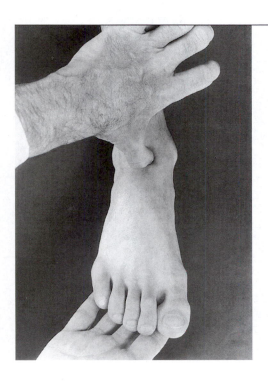

### FIGURE 11-57
### THE ANTERIOR BORDER OF THE LOWER EXTREMITY OF THE TIBIA

*Comment:*     *It is this border that is embedded in the transverse groove of the superior surface of the neck of the talus during dorsiflexion of the ankle.*

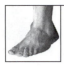

# THE POSTERIOR SURFACE OF THE ANKLE AND OF THE FOOT

The bony structures accessible by palpation are as follows:

- the medial malleolus (Fig. 11-59)
- the lesser process of the calcaneus (Fig. 11-60)
- the posterior surface of the calcaneus (Fig. 11-61)

- the posterior segment of the superior surface of the calcaneus (Fig. 11-62)
- the lateral malleolus (Fig. 11-63)
- the peroneal tubercle (Fig. 11-64)

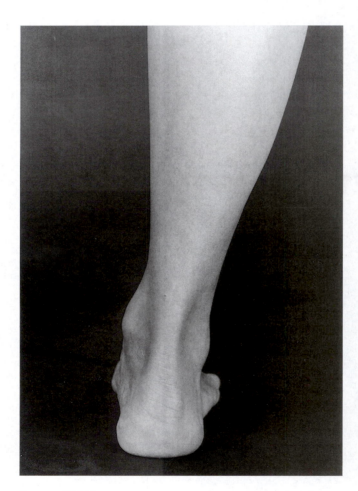

**FIGURE 11-58**
**POSTERIOR VIEW OF THE ANKLE AND OF THE FOOT**

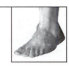

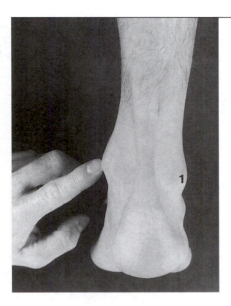

### FIGURE 11-59
### THE MEDIAL MALLEOLUS

This structure, indicated by the index finger, was also located during the approach to the medial border of the foot. This is a different view, which underlines its topography in relation to the other anatomic structures of the region.

*Comment:* **In this figure, the relatively high position of the medial malleolus in relation to the lateral malleolus (1) is clearly shown.**

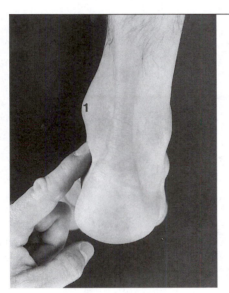

### FIGURE 11-60
### THE SUSTENTACULUM TALI

This structure, indicated by the index finger, was also discussed during the examination of the medial border of the foot. This posterior view confirms its topography in relation to the medial malleolus (1), approximately one fingerbreadth below.

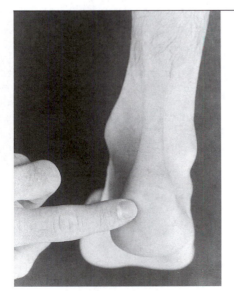

### FIGURE 11-61
### THE POSTERIOR SURFACE OF THE CALCANEUS

Narrow and smooth in its upper portion, this structure is wide and rough in its lower portion, where the Achilles tendon is attached. It is globally perceived under the fingers as triangular in shape with a wide inferior base.

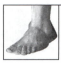

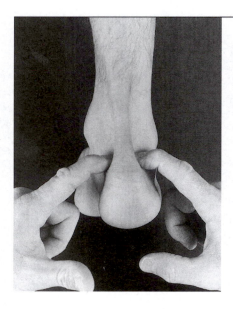

### FIGURE 11-62
### THE POSTERIOR SEGMENT OF THE SUPERIOR SURFACE OF THE CALCANEUS

Concave in the sagittal plane and convex in the transverse plane, this segment is approached on each side of the Achilles tendon.

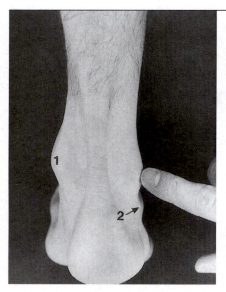

### FIGURE 11-63
### THE LATERAL MALLEOLUS

Indicated by the index finger, this structure was discussed during the examination of the lateral border of the foot. This different view emphasizes its relatively low position in relation to the medial malleolus (1) as well as its position in relation to the peroneal trochlea (2) (see Fig. 11-64).

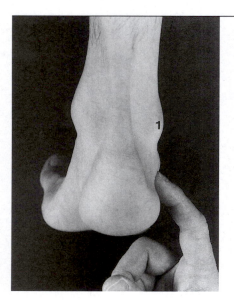

### FIGURE 11-64
### THE PERONEAL TROCHLEA

This structure was also discussed during the examination of the lateral border of the foot. This view stresses its position in relation to the apex of the lateral malleolus (1), which is approximately one fingerbreadth above.

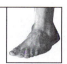

# THE PLANTAR SURFACE

The bony structures accessible by palpation are as follows:

- the heads of the five metatarsal bones (plantar view) (Fig. 11-66)
- the plantar surface of the cuboid bone (Fig. 11-67)
- the medial and lateral sesamoid bones (Figs. 11-68 and 11-69)
- the posterolateral tubercle of the first metatarsal bone (Fig. 11-70)
- the anterior tuberosity of the inferior surface of the calcaneus (plantar view) (Fig. 11-71)

- the posterior segment of the inferior surface of the calcaneus (Fig. 11-72)
- the posteromedial tubercle or tuberosity of the calcaneus (Fig. 11-73)
- the posterolateral tubercle or tuberosity of the calcaneus (Fig. 11-74)

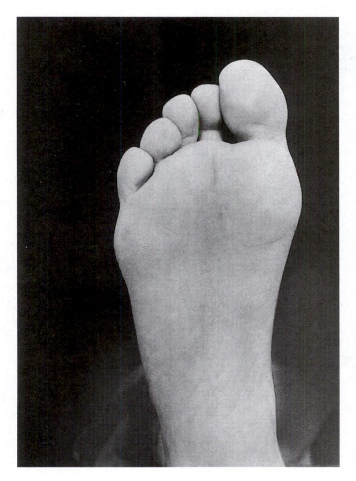

**FIGURE 11-65**
**PLANTAR VIEW OF THE FOOT**

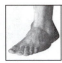

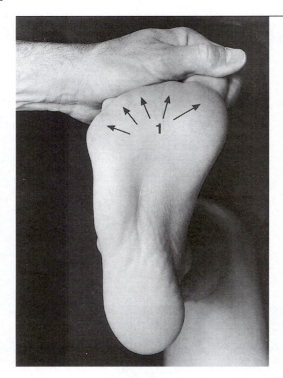

### FIGURE 11-66
#### THE HEADS OF THE FIVE METATARSAL BONES—PLANTAR VIEW

A characteristic of each metatarsal bone is that the head is covered by a convex articular surface that extends more on the plantar side than on the dorsal side.

This characteristic is recognized during palpation by finding a wide convex and smooth surface under the fingers (1) just behind the metatarsophalangeal joint of each of the five metatarsal bones.

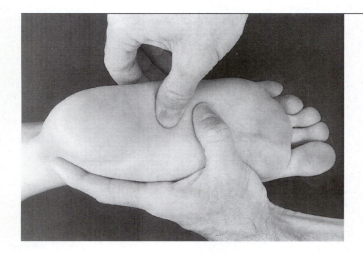

### FIGURE 11-67
#### THE PLANTAR SURFACE OF THE CUBOID BONE

This bone was already studied during the examination of the lateral border of the foot. After locating the tuberosity of the fifth metatarsal bone (Figs. 11-7 and 11-8) and the greater process of the calcaneus (Figs. 11-7 and 11-13), the thumb is placed between the two structures mentioned and slides around the lateral border of the foot and the lateral border of the cuboid bone (Fig. 11-9). It is now positioned on the plantar surface of this bone.

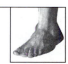

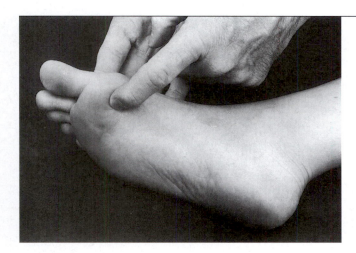

### FIGURE 11-68
### THE MEDIAL SESAMOID BONE

Place a digital grip on the plantar surface of the head of the first metatarsal bone and proceed with a transverse friction. This technique allows the perception under the finger of two "tubercles" separated by a depression.

In this picture, the index finger hooks up the medial sesamoid bone.

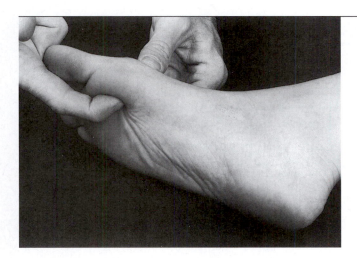

### FIGURE 11-69
### THE LATERAL SESAMOID BONE

The technique here is the same as that described in Fig. 11-68. The index finger is placed toward the lateral border of the foot to perceive (just beyond the depression mentioned) the lateral sesamoid bone.

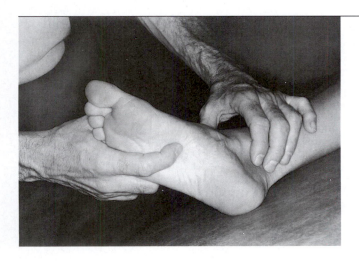

### FIGURE 11-70
### THE POSTEROLATERAL TUBERCLE OF THE FIRST METATARSAL BONE

After locating the base of the first metatarsal bone, move to the plantar surface of the foot toward the lateral border (this picture shows its position) (see also Fig. 11-34).

*Comment:*     *Since this structure is deeply located, the application of a reasonably firm pressure is recommended in order to have access to it. An approach using the thumb might prove more effective.*

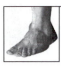

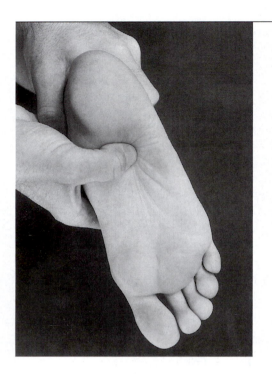

### FIGURE 11-71
### THE ANTERIOR TUBERCLE OF THE INFERIOR SURFACE OF THE CALCANEUS

This figure presents a plantar view of the foot, which allows a more precise identification of the topographic position of the examined structure.

If the approach is carried from the medial border, the neck of the talus (Figs. 11-32 and 11-41) serves as a landmark when the thumb is placed at its level. Afterwards, the fingers move around the medial border of the foot in order to find the investigated structure.

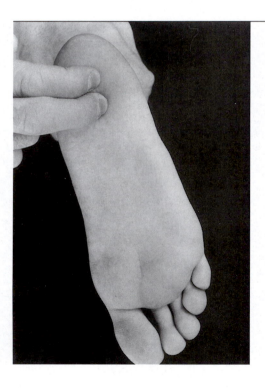

### FIGURE 11-72
### THE POSTERIOR SEGMENT OF THE INFERIOR SURFACE OF THE CALCANEUS

Also designated as the posterior tuberosity, this structure occupies the posterior third of the bone and represents the part of the calcaneus lying on the ground (Fig. 11-7).

It presents two tubercles: the medial process (Fig. 11-73) and the lateral process (Fig. 11-74).

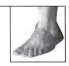

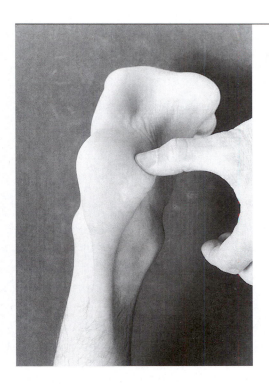

### FIGURE 11-73
### THE MEDIAL PROCESS

This is the largest of the two posterior tuberosities. It is the site of insertion of the flexor digitorum brevis and abductor hallucis muscles.

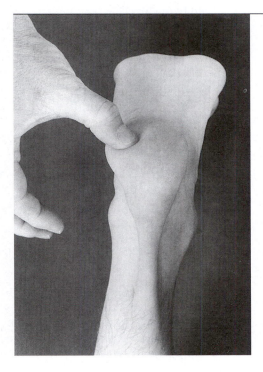

### FIGURE 11-74
### THE LATERAL PROCESS

This is the smallest of the two posterior tuberosities. It is the site of insertion of the abductor digiti minimi muscle.

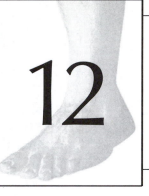

# 12

# ARTHROLOGY

## THE ARTICULATIONS

## THE ARTICULAR INTERSPACES AND THE LIGAMENTS

The articulations accessible during the surface investigation are (from the extremity of the toes to the ankle) as follows:

- the interphalangeal joints (Figs. 12-2 and 12-3)
- the metatarsophalangeal joints (Figs. 12-4, 12-5, and 12-6)
- the tarsometatarsal joints (Lisfranc) (Figs. 12-7 through 12-11)
- the "medial tarsal" joint (Chopart's) (Figs. 12-12, 12-13, and 12-14), including the "Y" ligament (Fig. 12-13)

- the posterior calcaneotalar or subtalar joint and the anterior calcaneotalar joint (Figs. 12-15 and 12-16)
- the tibiotarsal joint (Figs. 12-17 through 12-22)
- the ligaments of the tibiotarsal joint (Figs. 12-23 through 12-28)
- the posteroinferior tibiofibular ligament (Fig. 12-29)
- the lateral annular ligament tarsi (Fig. 12-30)
- the anterosuperior and anteroinferior annular ligament tarsi (Fig. 12-31)
- the aponeurosis of the foot (Fig. 12-32)

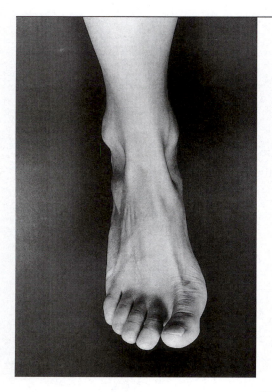

**FIGURE 12-1**

**ANTERIOR VIEW OF THE ANKLE AND DORSAL VIEW OF THE FOOT**

***Comment:*** ***The joint of Lisfranc (tarsometatarsal joints)***

This structure joins the three cuneiform bones and the cuboid bone to the five metatarsal bones. It includes three tarsometatarsal joints:

- a medial joint between the medial cuneiform bone and the first metatarsal bone
- an intermediate joint, which joins the middle and lateral cuneiform bones to the second and third metatarsal bones
- a lateral joint between the cuboid bone and the fourth and fifth metatarsal bones

The articulation of Chopart (medial tarsal joint) joins the distal tarsum to the proximal tarsum. From a functional point of view, it is a single unit that includes the calcaneotalonavicular joint and the calcaneocuboid joint. The "Y" ligament of Chopart is the ligament shared by the two articulations mentioned above.

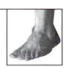

# THE INTERPHALANGEAL JOINTS

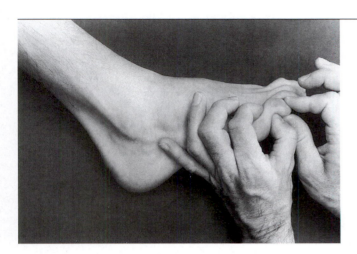

### FIGURE 12-2
#### THE INTERPHALANGEAL JOINTS OF THE FIFTH TOE

There are two of these and they can be identified without difficulty.

In this figure, the proximal grip immobilizes the proximal phalanx while the distal grip brings the distal phalanx into plantarflexion.

*Comment:* *These are trochlear joints (ginglymus). The opposing surfaces are the articular surface of the anterior extremity of the more posterior phalanx, which has the shape of a pulley, and the articular surface of the posterior extremity of the more anterior phalanx, which has a minimally pronounced middle ridge.*

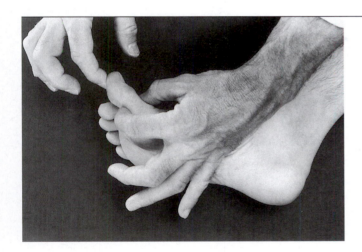

### FIGURE 12-3
#### THE INTERPHALANGEAL JOINT OF THE FIRST TOE
#### IN DORSAL EXTENSION

At the level of the first toe there is only one interphalangeal joint. In this figure, the proximal grip immobilizes the proximal phalanx while the distal grip brings the second phalanx into extension.

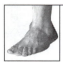
# THE METATARSOPHALANGEAL JOINTS

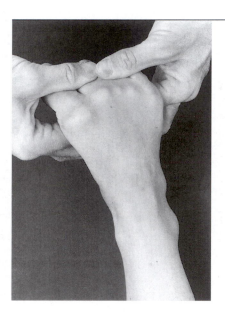

### FIGURE 12-4
#### THE METATARSOPHALANGEAL JOINTS—DORSAL VIEW

In this figure, the two hands grab the toes and bring them into plantarflexion, thereby uncovering the anterior and dorsal articular surfaces of the metatarsal heads.

*Comment:* *The articular surface is perceived under the fingers as a smooth surface. The most accessible is obviously that of the first toe.*

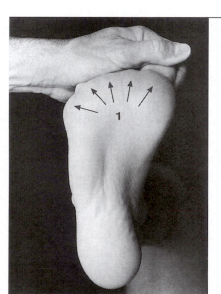

### FIGURE 12-5
#### THE METATARSOPHALANGEAL JOINTS—PLANTAR VIEW

In this picture, the hand grabs the toes and brings them into dorsiflexion, thereby uncovering the anterior and plantar articular surfaces of the metatarsal heads (1).

*Comment:* *The articular surface of the head of each metatarsal bone extends widely on the plantar side.*

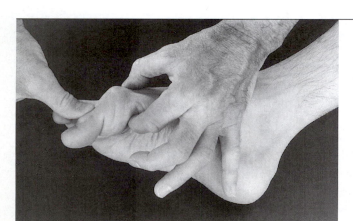

### FIGURE 12-6
#### THE METATARSOPHALANGEAL JOINT OF THE FIRST TOE

When this joint is examined, the sesamoid bones are palpated on its plantar portion (see Figs. 11-68 and 11-69).

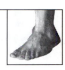

# THE ARTICULATION OF LISFRANC OR THE TARSOMETATARSAL JOINTS

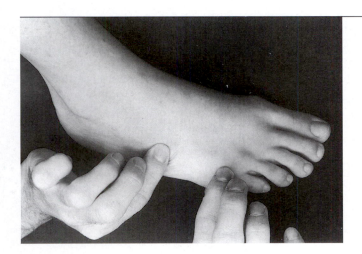

## FIGURE 12-7

### THE ARTICULAR INTERSPACE BETWEEN THE CUBOID BONE AND THE FIFTH METATARSAL BONE

The index finger of the distal hand is positioned on the anterior and lateral portion of the cuboid bone (Figs. 11-7, 11-9, 11-10, and 11-11) and the base of the fifth metatarsal bone (Figs. 11-7 and 11-8). To perceive the articular interspace, grab the head of the fifth metatarsal bone and mobilize it downward and then upward in a repetitive manner, allowing the index finger to perceive the investigated interspace clearly.

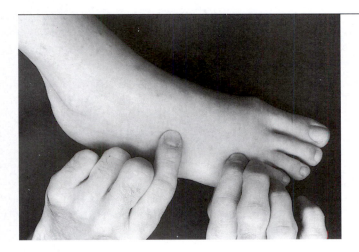

## FIGURE 12-8

### THE ARTICULAR INTERSPACE BETWEEN THE CUBOID BONE AND THE FOURTH METATARSAL BONE

While in contact with the base of the fourth metatarsal bone, move slightly inward the index finger of the proximal hand to face the anterior and medial portions of the cuboid bone.

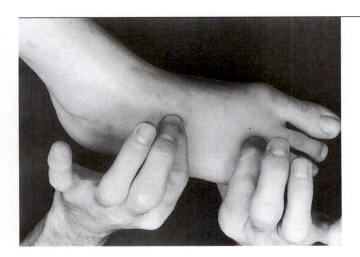

## FIGURE 12-9

### THE ARTICULAR INTERSPACE BETWEEN THE LATERAL CUNEIFORM BONE AND THE THIRD METATARSAL BONE

From the grip described above, the index finger moves approximately one fingerbreadth toward the medial aspect of the foot in order to be in contact with both the anterior border of the lateral cuneiform bone and the base of the third metatarsal bone.

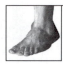

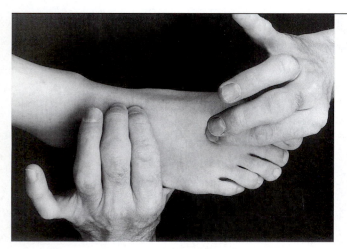

### FIGURE 12-10

**THE ARTICULAR INTERSPACE BETWEEN THE INTERMEDIATE CUNEIFORM BONE AND THE SECOND METATARSAL BONE**

Using the previous grip (Fig. 12-9), move by approximately one fingerbreadth toward the medial aspect of the foot, keeping in mind that the anterior border of the middle cuneiform bone is withdrawn in relation to the anterior border of the two surrounding cuneiform bones. This will displace the index finger toward the posterior aspect of the foot in order to be in contact with the middle cuneiform bone and the base of the second metatarsal bone.

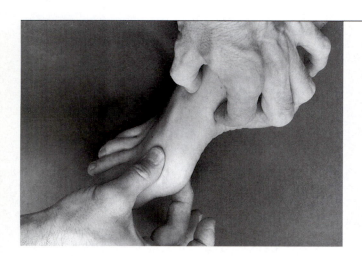

### FIGURE 12-11

**THE ARTICULAR INTERSPACE BETWEEN THE MEDIAL CUNEIFORM BONE AND THE FIRST METATARSAL BONE**

In this picture, to locate the medial cuneiform bone (see Figs. 11-7 and 11-32) the proximal grip is positioned at the level of the investigated interspace. The distal grip mobilizes the head of the first metatarsal bone.

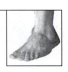

# THE ARTICULATION OF CHOPART OR THE MEDIAL TARSAL JOINT

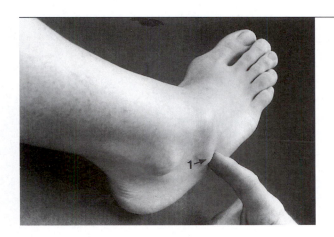

**FIGURE 12-12**

**THE LATERAL COMPONENT OF THE MEDIAL TARSAL JOINT ("LATERAL CHOPART")**

The index finger is placed on the cuboid facet of the calcaneus. This facet corresponds to the anterior surface of the calcaneus. It articulates in front with the cuboid bone.

A foot inversion facilitates access to the lateral portion of this surface. (1) Greater process of the calcaneus.

See comment on page 54.

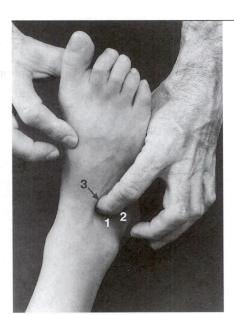

**FIGURE 12-13**

**THE "Y" LIGAMENT OF THE MEDIAL TARSAL JOINT**

This ligament attaches posteriorly to the dorsal surface of the greater process of the calcaneus (1). It divides into two bundles:

- a lateral bundle, which inserts into the dorsal surface of the cuboid bone (2)
- a medial bundle, which inserts into the entire height of the lateral surface of the navicular bone (3)

*Comment:*    *It is considered the key ligament of the joint being discussed.*

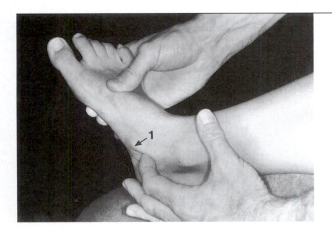

**FIGURE 12-14**

**THE MEDIAL ASPECT OF THE MEDIAL TARSAL JOINT ("MEDIAL CHOPART")**

An eversion of the foot allows a clearing of the head of the talus, which articulates anteriorly with the navicular bone (1).

In this figure, the index finger faces the middle field of the head of the talus, which corresponds to the inferior calcaneonavicular ligament. This smooth surface is perceived beneath the index finger.

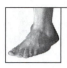

# THE POSTERIOR CALCANEOTALAR OR SUBTALAR JOINT AND THE ANTERIOR CALCANEOTALAR JOINT

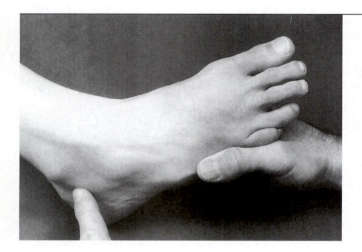

## FIGURE 12-15

### THE POSTERIOR CALCANEOTALAR OR SUBTALAR JOINT: LATERAL VIEW

The index finger indicates the lateral interspace of the subtalar joint. The bony prominence, facing the index finger, is the lateral process of the talus, which supports the most lateral portion of the peroneal facet of the body of the talus.

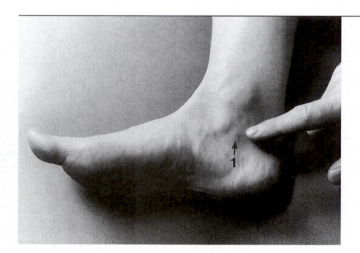

## FIGURE 12-16

### THE ANTERIOR CALCANEOTALAR JOINT: MEDIAL VIEW

The index finger indicates the medial interspace of the subtalar joint. The bony prominence facing the index finger is the lesser process of the calcaneus (1). It supports the intermediate articular surface of the calcaneus and constitutes a combined articular body, since it is in continuity with the anterior articular surface.

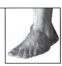

# THE TIBIOTARSAL JOINT

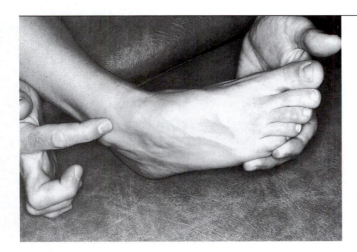

### FIGURE 12-17

### THE LATERAL BORDER OF THE LATERAL ASPECT OF THE TALAR TROCHLEA

The index finger of the distal hand is placed on the anterior border of the lower extremity of the peroneal shaft, while the foot is in neutral position. The foot may be slightly plantarflexed in order to perceive the investigated border under the finger.

The addition of a slight adduction of the foot may sharpen this perception.

*Comment:*     *Although smooth (since covered by cartilage), this border is perceived as sharp.*

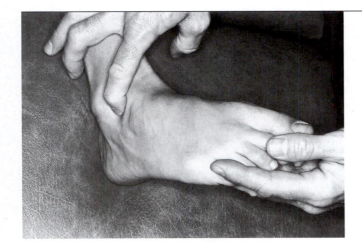

### FIGURE 12-18

### THE PERONEAL OR LATERAL MALLEOLAR FACET

With the subject's foot in neutral position, place the index finger of your proximal hand in front of the anterior border of the lower extremity of the fibula. With the distal hand, the foot is inverted and a slight plantarflexion is added. The articular facet is then perceived under the index finger as a smooth surface.

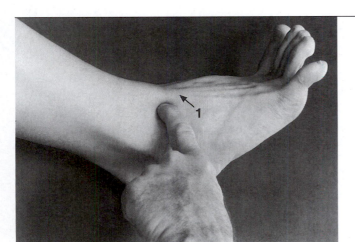

### FIGURE 12-19

### THE LATERAL ASPECT OF THE TALAR TROCHLEA

From the already located lateral border (Fig. 12-17), slide your finger behind the tendon of the extensor digitorum longus muscle (1) toward the medial border of the foot.

By inverting and plantarflexing the foot (projecting the talar trochlea toward the lateral aspect of the foot), access to this articular structure will be facilitated.

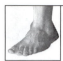

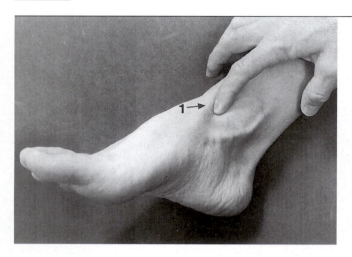

## Figure 12-20
### The medial border of the medial aspect of the talar trochlea

With the subject's foot in neutral position, the index finger of your distal hand is positioned on the anterior border of the medial malleolus, at its junction with the anterior border of the lower extremity of the tibial shaft.

Slightly plantarflex the foot in order to perceive the investigated border under the finger. It is preferable to add a slight eversion of the foot so that the examination will not be hampered by the tendon of the anterior tibialis muscle (1).

Comment:    *This border, perceived as a smooth structure beneath the finger, is much less pronounced on the medial side.*

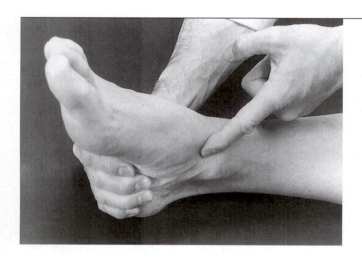

## Figure 12-21
### The tibial or medial malleolar facet

After placing the index finger of the distal hand in front of the anterior border of the medial malleolus, invert and slightly plantarflex the foot in order to expose the tibial facet optimally.

The investigated articular surface is perceived as a smooth surface beneath the finger.

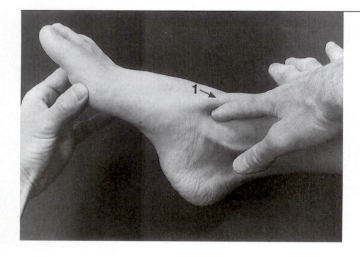

## Figure 12-22
### The medial aspect of the talar trochlea

From the already located medial border (Fig. 12-20), slide your fingers behind the tendon of the anterior tibialis muscle (1) toward the lateral border of the foot.

From this initial position, evert and plantarflex the foot in order to project the talar trochlea over the medial border of the foot. This will facilitate access to the investigated articular structure.

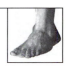

# THE LIGAMENTS OF THE TIBIOTARSAL JOINT

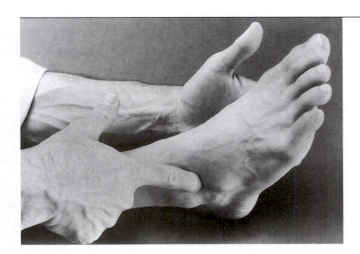

## FIGURE 12-23
### THE ANTERIOR TALOFIBULAR LIGAMENT

To approach this ligament, remember its proximal insertion (into the middle aspect of the anterior border of the lateral malleolus) and its distal insertion (into the talus) just in front of the peroneal facet.

It is sometimes useful to bring the foot into adduction, supination, and slight plantarflexion in order to better access this ligamentous structure.

Comment:    *These three ligaments (Figs. 12-23, 12-24, and 12-25) are part of the lateral lateral ligament.*

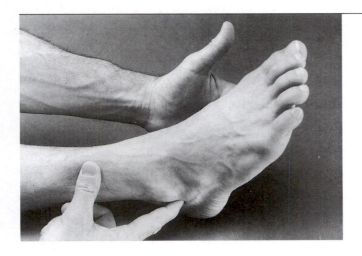

## FIGURE 12-24
### THE CALCANEOFIBULAR LIGAMENT

To properly study this ligamentous structure, its course as well as its proximal insertion (into the anterior border of the lateral malleolus, under the ligament described in Fig. 12-23) and distal insertion (into the lateral surface of the calcaneus) must be well visualized.

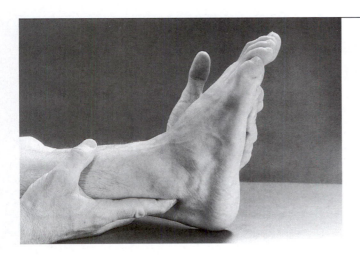

## FIGURE 12-25
### THE POSTERIOR TALOFIBULAR LIGAMENT

To localize this structure, it is essential to remember its lateral insertion (into the medial surface of the lateral malleolus, below and behind its articular surface) as well its medial insertion (into the lateral process of the posterior border of the talus).

Running between these two bony structures, its course is essentially horizontal.

Comment:    *It is located below the posterior inferior tibiofibular ligament of the inferior tibiofibular joint.*

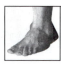

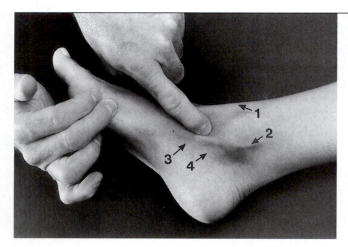

### FIGURE 12-26
### THE SUPERFICIAL LAYER OF THE DELTOID LIGAMENT:
### THE TIBIONAVICULAR BUNDLE

To find this layer, remember the sites of proximal (anterior border and apex of the medial malleolus) and distal insertion [superior surface of the navicular bone; medial surface of the neck of the talus; inferior calcaneonavicular ligament (3), and lesser process of the calcaneus (4)].

The simultaneous placement under tension of the tendons of the anterior tibialis muscle (1) and posterior tibialis muscle (2) (see figure) allows for localization of the most anterior part of this superficial layer, indicated by the index finger.

*Comment:* *When the tibionavicular bundle of the medial lateral ligament is palpated, you are also in contact with the anterior talotibial bundle of the deep layer of this ligament.*

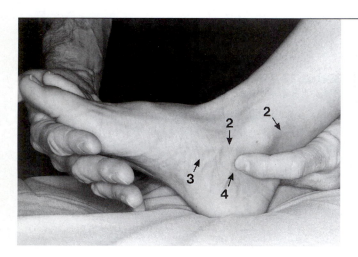

### FIGURE 12-27
### THE SUPERFICIAL LAYER OF THE DELTOID LIGAMENT:
### THE CALCANEOTIBIAL BUNDLE

This part of the ligament, which attaches to the inferior calcaneonavicular ligament (3), is approached below the tendon of the posterior tibialis muscle (2).

In this figure, it is the most posterior part of the superficial layer of the approached ligament (the one inserting into the lesser process of the calcaneus) (4).

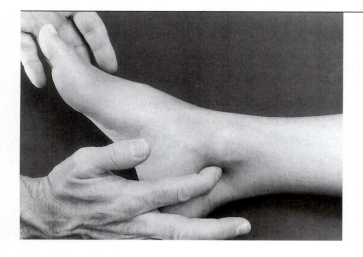

### FIGURE 12-28
### THE DEEP LAYER OF THE DELTOID LIGAMENT—THE POSTERIOR
### TALOTIBIAL BUNDLE

It is important to remember its slightly withdrawn tibial insertion into the apex of the medial malleolus (closer to the talus than the insertions of the superficial layer) and its insertion into the talus on the medial process. The fibers of the deep layer are stretched between these two structures.

*Comment:* *This region should be approached with care, since it is the site of passage of the posterior tibial artery and nerve.*

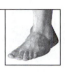

# THE POSTEROINFERIOR TIBIOFIBULAR LIGAMENT

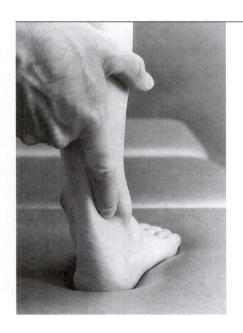

**FIGURE 12-29**
**THE POSTEROINFERIOR TIBIOFIBULAR LIGAMENT**

When the index finger slides into the lateral retromalleolar groove, the first ligament perceived under the finger (moving inferiorly) is the posteroinferior tibiofibular ligament. Below this ligament, one finds a bundle of fibers reinforcing the articular capsule and, finally, lower down, one contacts the posterior talofibular ligament which is the posterior bundle of the lateral lateral ligament.

# THE ANNULAR LIGAMENTS OF THE TARSUM AND THE DORSAL APONEUROSIS OF THE FOOT

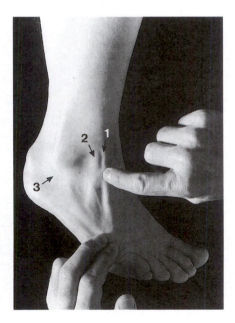

**FIGURE 12-30**
**THE LATERAL ANNULAR LIGAMENT OF THE TARSUM**

In this figure, the index finger clearly indicates the visualized lateral portion of the anterior annular ligaments of the tarsum, which cover the tendons of the extensor digitorum longus (1) and the peroneus tertius muscles (2) and extend to the lateral border of the foot by the lateral annular ligament of the tarsum (3).

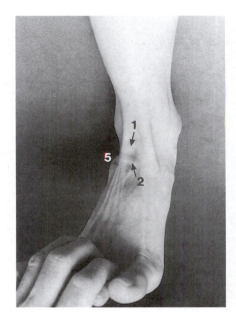

**FIGURE 12-31**
**THE ANTEROSUPERIOR AND ANTEROINFERIOR ANNULAR LIGAMENTS OF THE TARSUM**

At the point where they separate, just after covering the extensor digitorum longus muscle (5), you can clearly visualize the anterosuperior annular ligament of the tarsum (1) as well as the anteroinferior annular ligament of the tarsum (2).

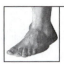

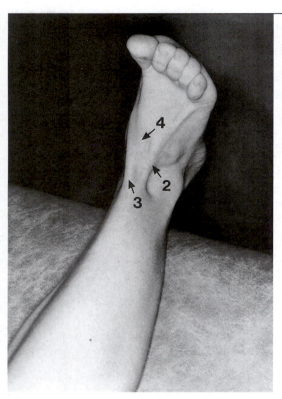

## FIGURE 12-32
### THE DORSAL APONEUROSIS OF THE FOOT

In this picture, you see clearly the dorsal aponeurosis of the foot (2), which covers the tendons of the extensor hallucis longus (4) and anterior tibialis muscles (3).

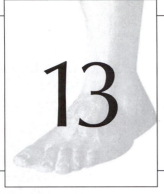

C H A P T E R

13

# MYOLOGY

## THE MUSCULOTENDINOUS STRUCTURES OF THE ANKLE AND THE FOOT

As you move around the ankle, you perceive the following:

- the tendon of the anterior tibialis muscle (Fig. 13-2)
- the tendon of the extensor hallucis longus muscle (Fig. 13-3)
- the extensor hallucis brevis muscle, integral part of the extensor digitorum brevis muscle (Figs. 13-4 and 13-7)
- the tendon of the extensor digitorum longus muscle (Fig. 13-5)
- the tendon of the peroneus tertius muscle (Fig. 13-6)
- the muscular body of the extensor digitorum brevis muscle (Fig. 13-7)
- the tendon of the peroneus brevis muscle (Fig. 13-8)
- the tendon of the peroneus longus muscle (Fig. 13-9)

- the posterior part of the muscular body of the peroneus brevis muscle (Fig. 13-10)
- the Achilles tendon (Figs. 13-11 and 13-12)
- the tendon of the posterior tibialis muscle at the level of the medial malleolus (Fig. 13-13)
- the tendon of the posterior tibialis muscle over the medial border of the foot (Fig. 13-14)
- the tendon of the flexor digitorum longus muscle at the level of the medial malleolus (Fig. 13-15)
- the tendon of the flexor digitorum longus muscle over the medial border of the foot (Fig. 13-16)
- the tendon of the flexor hallucis longus muscle in the medial retromalleolar groove (Fig. 13-17)
- the tendon of the flexor hallucis longus muscle over the medial border of the foot (Fig. 13-18)

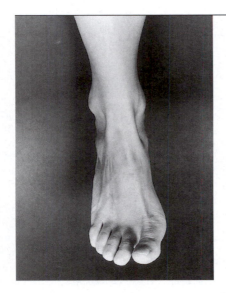

**FIGURE 13-1**
**ANTERIOR VIEW OF THE ANKLE AND DORSAL VIEW OF THE FOOT**

*Comment:*    *The presentation of this topographic region should not be considered in its strict sense. It is only a didactic means of approaching structures that extend to the level of the foot.*

177

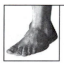

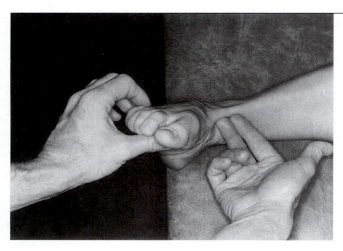

## FIGURE 13-2
### THE TENDON OF THE ANTERIOR TIBIALIS MUSCLE

A large, powerful tendon, which has the shape of a cylindrical cord, appears in front of the medial malleolus, extending toward the medial border of the foot, where its principal site of insertion is the medial cuneiform bone. In this picture, the proximal hand positions the foot in inversion and dorsiflexion. The subject is asked to maintain this position.

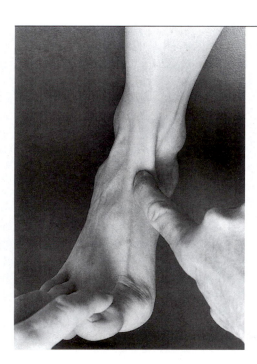

## FIGURE 13-3
### THE TENDON OF THE EXTENSOR HALLUCIS LONGUS MUSCLE

Ask the subject to perform a double extension at the level of the interphalangeal and metatarsophalangeal joints of the first toe. A resistance may be applied by the thumb to the dorsal aspect of the first toe in order to sensitize the subject to the movement requested. The tendon appears just lateral to the tendon of the anterior tibialis muscle.

*Comment:*    *The tendon of this muscle also participates in the adduction, supination, and dorsiflexion of the ankle.*

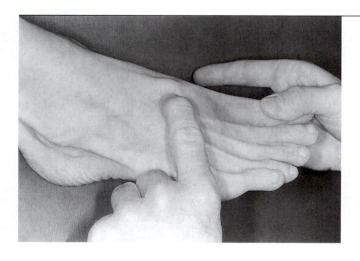

## FIGURE 13-4
### THE MUSCULAR BODY OF THE EXTENSOR HALLUCIS BREVIS MUSCLE

Since it is the muscular head intended for the first toe, this body inconsistently constitutes the medialmost portion of the extensor digitorum brevis muscle.

Have the subject perform repeated extensions of the metatarsophalangeal joint of the first toe to assist in locating it on the dorsum of the foot, just lateral to the tendon of the extensor digitorum longus muscle, as located in Fig. 13-3.

*Comment:*    *Its access is not easy and there are very few subjects in whom it is approached without difficulty (see also Fig. 13-23).*

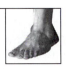

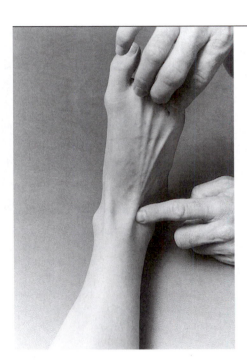

## Figure 13-5
### The tendon of the extensor digitorum longus muscle

This muscle participates in dorsiflexion of the ankle. The subject should therefore be asked to perform this muscular action in order to demonstrate the tendon at the level of the ankle, just lateral to the tendon of the extensor hallucis longus muscle (Fig. 13-4).

A resistance globally applied to the dorsal surface of the phalanges of the last four toes (against the extension of the interphalangeal and metatarsophalangeal joints of these toes) results in the demonstration of the tendons on the dorsum of the foot.

*Comment:* ***This muscle also participates in the abduction, pronation, and dorsiflexion of the foot.***

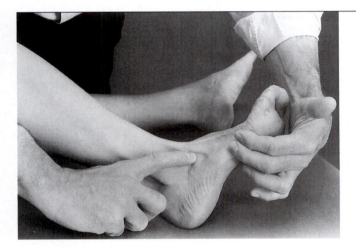

## Figure 13-6
### The tendon of the peroneus tertius muscle

The subject is asked to abduct, pronate, and dorsiflex the foot against resistance as a grip is positioned on the lateral border of the foot, as shown in this picture.

The tendon appears lateral to the tendon of the extensor digitorum longus muscle, intended for the fifth toe. It extends toward the dorsal surface of the base of the fifth metatarsal bone, which is its site of distal insertion.

*Comment:* ***It is not constant.***

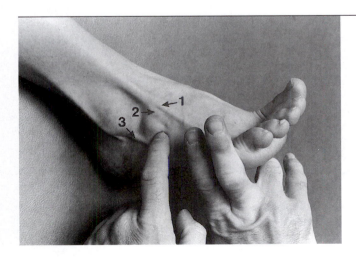

## Figure 13-7
### The muscular body of the extensor digitorum brevis muscle

The subject is asked to perform an extension of the interphalangeal and metatarsophalangeal joints of the toes in a global fashion (the fifth toe is not involved with this muscle).

The muscular body appears lateral to the tendons of the extensor digitorum longus muscle (1) and of the peroneus tertius muscle (2), in front of the lateral malleolus and medial to the tendon of the peroneus brevis muscle (3).

*Comment:* ***Resistance applied to the lateral border of the foot by the distal hand is intended to project the tendinous structures surrounding the investigated muscle, indicated by the index finger.***

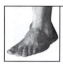

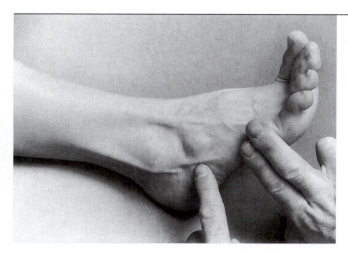

### FIGURE 13-8
### THE TENDON OF THE PERONEUS BREVIS MUSCLE

With the foot in neutral position, the subject is asked to perform a pure abduction of the foot.

The distal hand may offer resistance on the lateral border of the foot.

The index finger of the proximal hand indicates the investigated structure.

*Comment:     This tendon passes in front of the peroneal tubercle.*

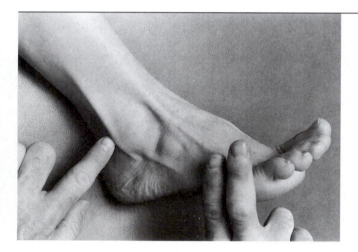

### FIGURE 13-9
### THE TENDON OF THE PERONEUS LONGUS MUSCLE

The subject is asked to perform the same movement described above. This might be sufficient to demonstrate the tendon over the lateral border of the foot just before its entrance into the groove of the cuboid bone. A pronation and a plantarflexion may be added.

*Comment:     This tendon passes behind the peroneal trochlea.*

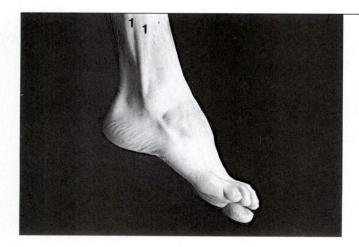

### FIGURE 13-10
### THE POSTERIOR PORTION OF THE MUSCULAR BODY OF THE PERONEUS BREVIS MUSCLE

The muscular action requested from the subject is the same as that described in Fig. 13-9.

The muscular body (1) is accessible slightly above the lateral malleolus and behind the tendon of the peroneus longus muscle.

In certain subjects (see figure), it may also be seen in front of this tendon.

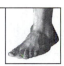

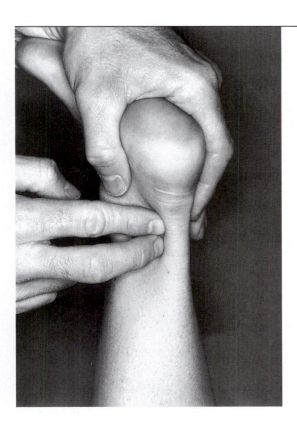

**FIGURE 13-11**
**LATERAL AND POSTERIOR APPROACH
TO THE ACHILLES TENDON**

This tendon, being superficial, does not present any difficulty of access.

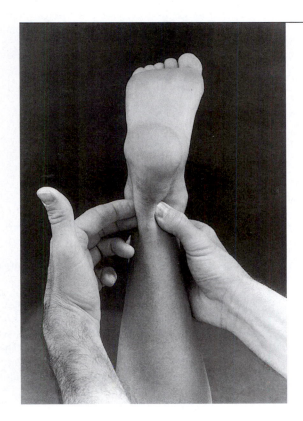

**FIGURE 13-12**

**THE ANTEROLATERAL AND ANTEROMEDIAL APPROACH
TO THE ACHILLES TENDON**

Using the thumb, push the tendon laterally in order to gain access to its anterolateral portion, which may be investigated through sliding (to-and-fro) digital movements. Similarly, push the tendon medially with the thumb in order to gain access to its anteromedial portion.

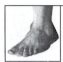

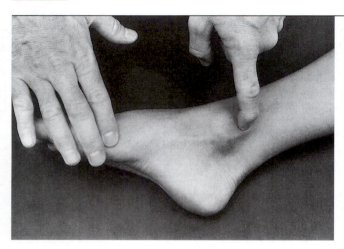

## FIGURE 13-13
### THE TENDON OF THE POSTERIOR TIBIALIS MUSCLE
### AT THE LEVEL OF THE MEDIAL MALLEOLUS

With the foot in plantarflexion, the subject is asked to adduct the foot against resistance over the medial border.

The tendon appears on the posterior border of the medial malleolus.

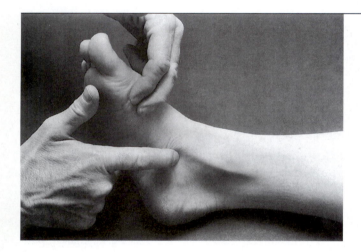

## FIGURE 13-14
### THE TENDON OF THE POSTERIOR TIBIALIS MUSCLE

The technique of placing this tendon under tension is the same as that described above.

After passing around the medial malleolus, the tendon follows the medial border of the foot, where it inserts, among other bony structures, into the tubercle of the navicular bone, indicated by the index finger.

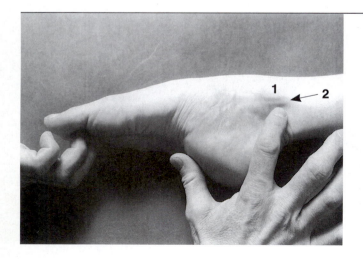

## FIGURE 13-15
### THE TENDON OF THE FLEXOR DIGITORUM LONGUS MUSCLE
### AT THE LEVEL OF THE MEDIAL MALLEOLUS

One hand is placed on the plantar surface of the last four toes in order to solicit repeated flexion of these toes. These repeated muscular actions are perceived by the other hand, which is positioned behind the posterior tibialis muscle (1). The index finger demonstrates the tendon of the flexor digitorum longus muscle (2), which is also situated behind the medial malleolus.

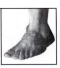

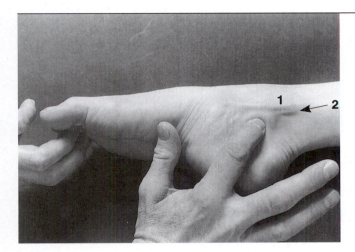

## Figure 13-16
### The tendon of the flexor digitorum longus muscle over the medial border of the foot

After passing around the medial malleolus in a special osteofibrous sheath, this tendon crosses the medial lateral ligament of the ankle joint and runs through its groove on the lesser process of the calcaneus. In this picture, the index finger is placed at the level of this groove. Beyond that, the tendon of the flexor digitorum longus muscle (2) extends into the plantar surface of the foot.

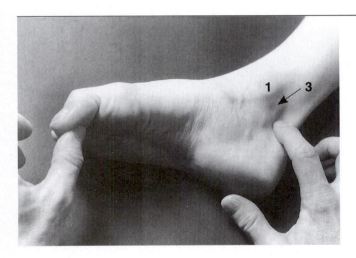

## Figure 13-17
### The tendon of the flexor hallucis longus muscle in the medial retromalleolar groove

One hand is positioned on the plantar surface of the first toe to solicit repeated flexions of the same toe.

These repeated muscular actions are perceived in the medial retromalleolar groove at some distance from the medial malleolus and very close to the Achilles tendon.

*Comment:*  *The tendon (3) of the investigated muscle, shown in this picture, is not visible in all patients.*

---

### Figures 13-16, 13-17, and 13-18

1.  Posterior tibialis muscle
2.  Flexor digitorum longus muscle
3.  Flexor hallucis longus muscle

---

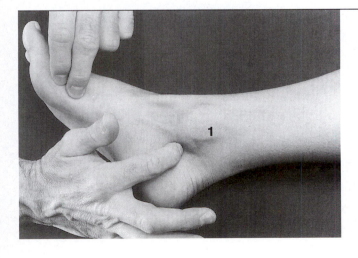

## Figure 13-18
### The tendon of the flexor hallucis longus muscle over the medial border of the foot

Beyond the tibiotarsal joint, the tendon slides into the groove of the posterior surface of the talus and positions itself under the tendon of the flexor digitorum longus muscle (Fig. 13-16) (2) in a special groove involving the medial surface of the calcaneus and located below the sustentaculum tali.

*Comment:*  *It may be interesting (as in this picture) to stress the tendon of the posterior tibialis muscle, since it is a landmark in the investigation of the examined tendon.*

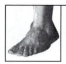

184 MYOLOGY

# THE INTRINSIC MUSCLES OF THE FOOT

The muscular structures accessible by palpation are as follows:

- the extensor digitorum brevis and the extensor hallucis brevis muscles (Figs. 13-21 and 13-25)
- the abductor digiti minimi muscle (Fig. 13-26)
- the flexor digiti minimi brevis muscle (Fig. 13-27)
- the opponens digiti minimi muscle: visualization of its action (Fig. 13-28)
- the abductor hallucis muscle (Fig. 13-29)

- the flexor hallucis brevis muscle (Fig. 13-30)
- the adductor hallucis muscle (Fig. 13-31)
- the quadratus plantae muscle: visualization of its action (Fig. 13-32)
- the flexor digitorum brevis muscle: visualization of its action (Fig. 13-33)
- the dorsal and plantar interossei muscles: visualization of their actions (Figs. 13-34, 13-35, and 13-36).

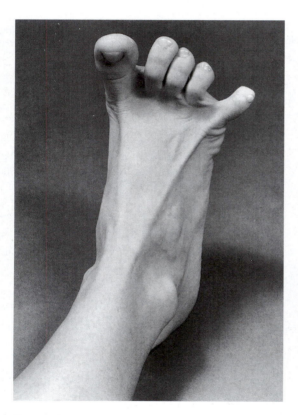

**FIGURE 13-19**
**DORSAL VIEW OF THE FOOT**

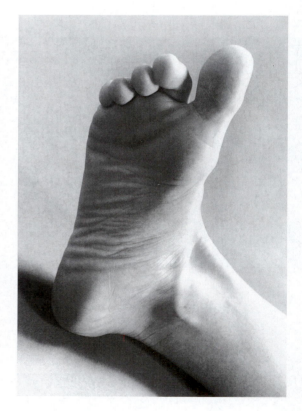

**FIGURE 13-20**
**PLANTAR VIEW OF THE FOOT**

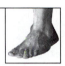

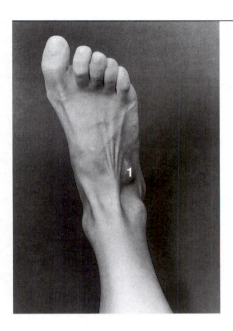

## FIGURE 13-21
### THE EXTENSOR DIGITORUM BREVIS MUSCLE—VISUALIZATION AND TOPOGRAPHY

This is the only muscle (1) in the dorsum of the foot.

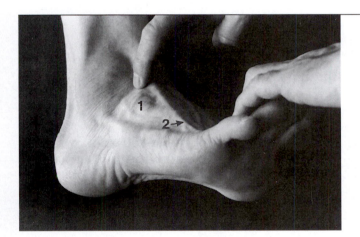

## FIGURE 13-22
### THE EXTENSOR DIGITORUM BREVIS MUSCLE

Ask the subject to perform an extension of the four proximal phalanges of the corresponding toes, with or without resistance, to perceive the muscular body (1), which is in front of the lateral malleolus and lateral to the tendon of the extensor digitorum longus muscle (2).

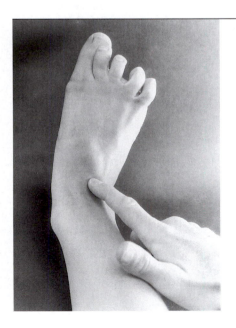

## FIGURE 13-23
### EXTENSOR HALLUCIS BREVIS MUSCLE

This is part of the extensor digitorum brevis muscle. The requested muscular action is the same as that described above. The muscular body is perceived in front of the anterior annular ligament of the tarsum (Figs. 12-31 and 12-32), lateral to the tendon of the extensor hallucis longus muscle (Fig. 13-4) and medial to the tendon of the extensor digitorum longus muscle (Fig. 13-6).

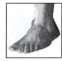

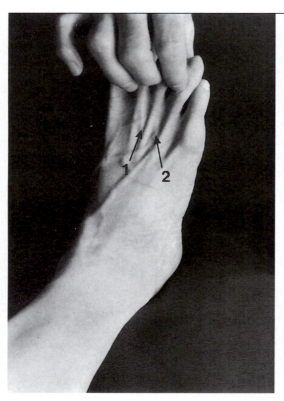

## FIGURE 13-24
### ENDING OF THE TENDONS OF THE EXTENSOR DIGITORUM BREVIS MUSCLE AT THE LEVEL OF THE SECOND AND THIRD TOES

The requested muscular action is the same as that described in Fig. 13-22. A digital grip placed on the dorsal surface of the toes brings these toes into plantarflexion in order to demonstrate the two tendons, ending at the tendons of the extensor digitorum longus muscle serving the second (1) and third toes (2).

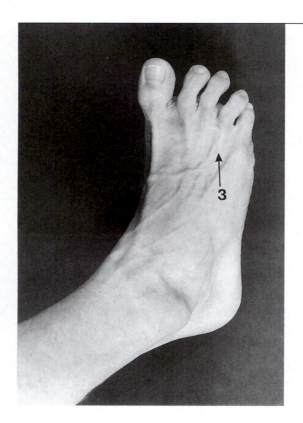

## FIGURE 13-25
### ENDING OF THE TENDON OF THE EXTENSOR DIGITORUM BREVIS MUSCLE AT THE LEVEL OF THE FOURTH TOE

This figure shows this tendon as it joins the tendon of the extensor digitorum longus muscle, serving the fourth toe (3).

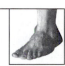

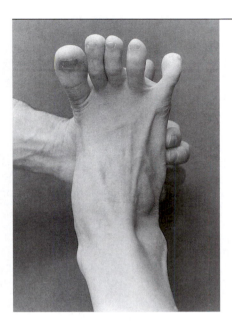

## FIGURE 13-26
### THE ABDUCTOR DIGITI MINIMI MUSCLE

Place a wide digital grip on the lateral border of the foot and the subject is asked for repeated abductions of the fifth toe. The muscular contraction is well perceived under the fingers.

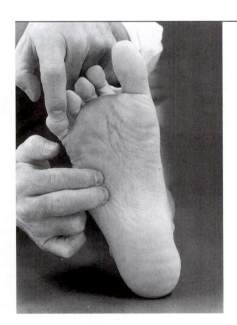

## FIGURE 13-27
### THE FLEXOR DIGITI MINIMI BREVIS MUSCLE

Position a bidigital grip on the plantar surface of the fifth metatarsal bone, moving slightly toward the medial border of the foot. Laterally, the muscular body is covered by the abductor digiti minimi muscle.

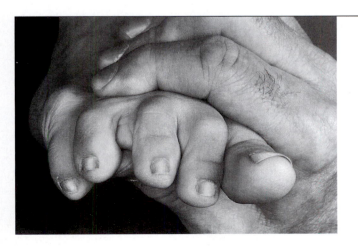

## FIGURE 13-28
### VISUALIZATION OF THE ACTION OF THE OPPONENS DIGITI MINIMI MUSCLE

Its action is to bring the fifth metatarsal bone medially.

*Comment:* *Like the two muscles mentioned above, this one belongs to the lateral muscular group. It cannot be palpated individually.*

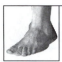

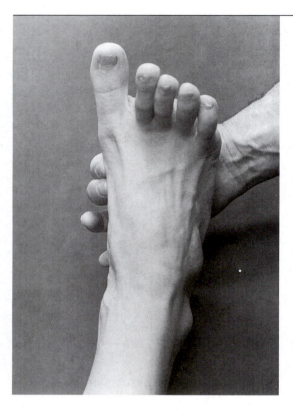

## FIGURE 13-29
### THE ABDUCTOR HALLUCIS MUSCLE

Place a wide digital grip on the medial border of the foot and the subject is asked to abduct the first toe on the first metatarsal bone.

If the subject cannot perform this type of muscular action, he or she should be asked to flex the first toe on the first metatarsal bone. The muscular contraction is well perceived on the medial border of the foot, more particularly on the plantar surface of the medial cuneiform bone and of the navicular bone.

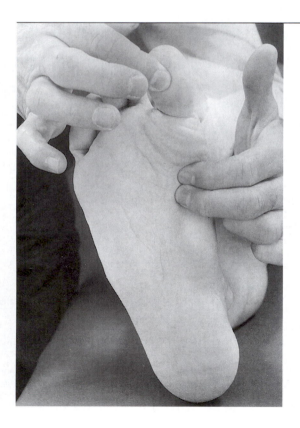

## FIGURE 13-30
### THE FLEXOR HALLUCIS BREVIS MUSCLE

Using a bidigital grip applied as widely as possible to the plantar surface of the first metatarsal bone behind the sesamoid bones, move slightly toward the medial border of the foot in order to perceive the medial bundle. For the lateral bundle, the grip should be moved toward the lateral border of the foot, keeping in mind that this bundle is partially covered by the tendon of the flexor hallucis longus muscle. The requested action is a flexion of the first toe on the first metatarsal bone.

*Comment:*    ***The superposition of the different muscular structures makes their individual palpation difficult.***

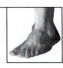

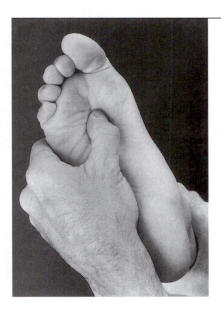

## FIGURE 13-31
### THE ADDUCTOR HALLUCIS MUSCLE

A wide grip using the thumb should be placed on the plantar surface of the first metatarsal interspace, with the hand placed on the lateral aspect of the foot. The subject is asked to flex the first toe at the first metatarsal bone in order to make the muscular contraction perceptible beneath the fingers. The contraction is perceived at the level of the oblique bundle and may be confused with the lateral bundle of the flexor hallucis brevis muscle. The perception of the contraction is difficult.

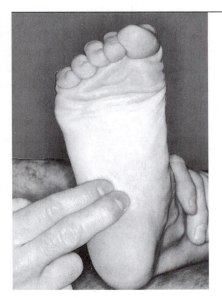

## FIGURE 13-32
### VISUALIZATION OF THE ACTION OF THE QUADRATUS PLANTAE MUSCLE

In this figure, the fingers are placed approximately at the junction of this muscle with the lateral border of the tendon of the flexor digitorum longus muscle.

*Comment:* *Because of its oblique course, the tendon of the flexor digitorum longus muscle creates a certain deviation of the foot and toes. The purpose of the investigated muscle is to correct this tendency.*

*Therefore, it participates in the flexion of the last four toes.*

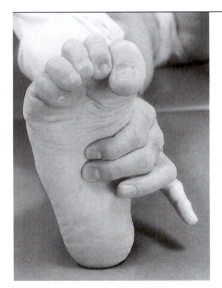

## FIGURE 13-33
### VISUALIZATION OF THE ACTION OF THE FLEXOR DIGITORUM BREVIS MUSCLE

A grip covering the foot through its medial or lateral border allows placement of a wide digital grip on the medial and plantar aspects of the foot.

Next, the subject is asked to perform repeated flexions of the toes on the metatarsal bones in order to make the muscular contraction perceptible beneath the fingers.

*Comment:* *The tendons described above are superposed on those of the flexor digitorum longus muscle.*

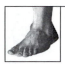

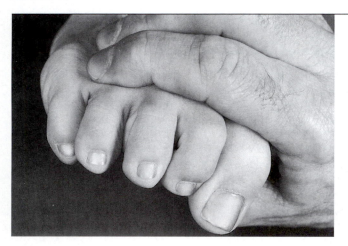

### FIGURE 13-34
### VISUALIZATION OF THE ACTION OF THE PLANTAR INTEROSSEI MUSCLES AND OF THE LUMBRICALES MUSCLES

This figure visualizes the flexion of the proximal phalanges on the metatarsal bones of the lateral four toes. Contrary to what is shown in the figure, the first toe is not involved in this action. The plantar interossei muscles flex the proximal phalanx of the lateral four toes and draw the last three toes into the axis of the foot (which passes through the second toe). The lumbricales muscles flex the proximal phalanx of the lateral four toes and extend the two distal phalanges on the proximal phalanx.

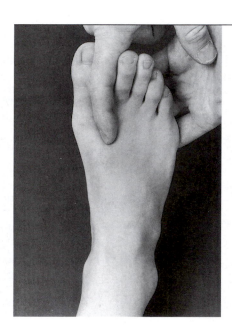

### FIGURE 13-35
### THE FIRST DORSAL INTEROSSEUS MUSCLE

The dorsal interossei muscles can be approached in the four metatarsal interspaces.

They are directly accessible beneath the fingers when they are placed against the medial and lateral surfaces of the metatarsal bones.

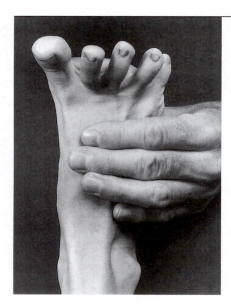

### FIGURE 13-36
### VISUALIZATION OF ONE OF THE PRINCIPAL ACTIONS OF THE DORSAL INTEROSSEI MUSCLES

In this figure, the primary action is that of abduction of the second, third, and fourth toes in relation to the axis of the foot (which passes through the second toe).

*Comment:* *These muscles also flex the proximal phalanx of the lateral four toes.*

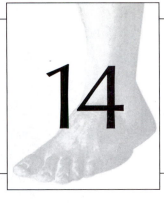

C H A P T E R

# 14

# NERVES AND VESSELS

The notable structures accessible by palpation are as follows:

- The musculocutaneous nerve (Figs. 14-3 and 14-4)
- the cutaneous lateral dorsal nerve (Fig. 14-4)
- the anastomosis between the cutaneous intermediate dorsal nerve and the cutaneous lateral dorsal nerve (Fig. 14-4)

- the cutaneous intermediate dorsal nerve (Fig. 14-5)
- the posterior tibial nerve (Figs. 14-7 and 14-8)
- the posterior tibial artery (Figs. 14-7 and 14-8)
- the dorsalis pedis artery (Fig. 14-9)

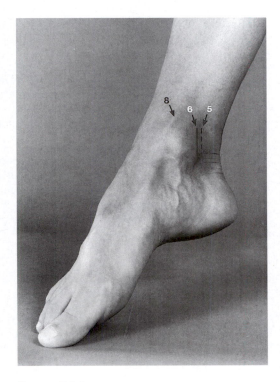

**FIGURE 14-1**

**MEDIAL VIEW OF THE ANKLE AND FOOT**

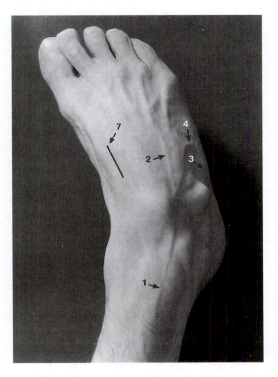

**FIGURE 14-2**

**ANTERIOR VIEW OF THE ANKLE AND DORSAL VIEW OF THE FOOT**

1. the superficial peroneal nerve
2. the cutaneous intermediate dorsal nerve
3. the cutaneous lateral dorsal nerve
4. the anastomosis between the cutaneous intermediate dorsal nerve and the cutaneous lateral dorsal nerve

5. the tibial nerve
6. the posterior tibial artery
7. the dorsalis pedis artery
8. the greater saphenous vein

191

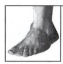

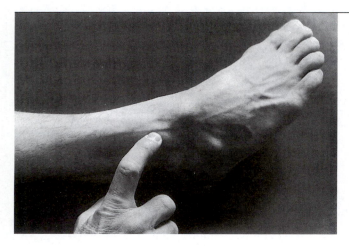

### Figure 14-3
### The superficial peroneal nerve

There are two possibilities for the investigation of this nerve:

- a relatively high search at the level of the inferior leg (at approximately the junction of the proximal two-thirds and of the distal third of the anterolateral aspect of the leg)
- a lower search at the level of the proximal foot

*Comment:* **In either case, the nerve runs subcutaneously after perforating the aponeurosis of the leg.**

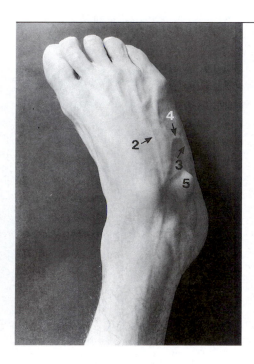

### Figure 14-4

### The cutaneous lateral dorsal nerve (3) and the anastomosis (4) between the cutaneous intermediate dorsal nerve (2) and the cutaneous lateral dorsal nerve (3)

In this figure, the musculocutaneous nerve is well visualized over the anterolateral and distal portion of the leg. At the level of the lateral malleolus, it extends through the cutaneous intermediate dorsal nerve (2), which travels along the third metatarsal interspace.

You can visualize the cutaneous lateral dorsal nerve (3), which is a prolongation of the sural nerve and travels along the lateral border of the foot. You can also see the anastomosis (4) between the two nerve structures described above, which passes just in front of the greater process of the calcaneus (5).

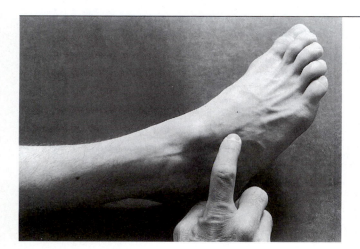

### Figure 14-5

### The cutaneous intermediate dorsal nerve

Lateral view: Its topographic relationship with the other nerve elements of this region are described above (Fig. 14-4).

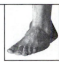

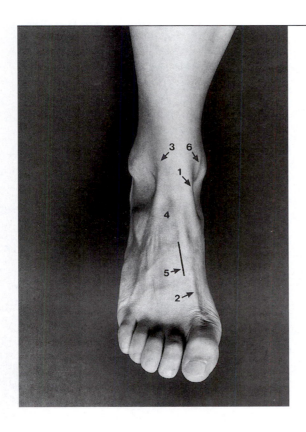

**FIGURE 14-6**
**ANTERIOR VIEW OF THE ANKLE AND OF THE FOOT**

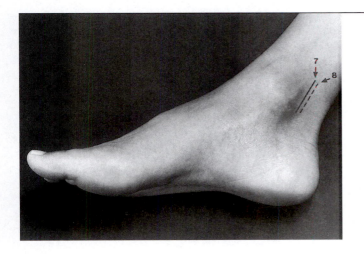

**FIGURE 14-7**
**MEDIAL VIEW OF THE ANKLE AND OF THE FOOT**

1. The tendon of the anterior tibialis muscle
2. The tendon of the extensor hallucis longus muscle
3. The tendon of the extensor digitorum longus muscle
4. The interior inferior annular ligament of the tarsum

5. The dorsalis pedis artery
6. The greater saphenous vein
7. The posterior tibial artery
8. The posterior tibial nerve

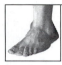 

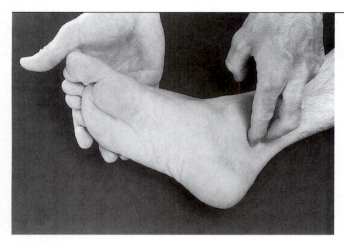

### FIGURE 14-8

### THE POSTERIOR TIBIAL ARTERY AND THE POSTERIOR TIBIAL NERVE

The artery enters the medial retromalleolar groove between the flexor digitorum longus muscle located anteriorly and the flexor hallucis longus muscle located posteriorly.

The examination of the pulse and, therefore, its localization will be facilitated if the foot is first placed in slight inversion in order to relax the soft tissues of the region.

The posterior tibial nerve is palpated just behind the artery as a full cylindrical cord.

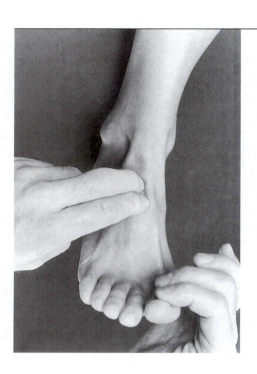

### FIGURE 14-9

### THE DORSALIS PEDIS ARTERY

This is the name given to the anterior tibial artery at the level of the anterior annular ligament of the tarsum (Figs. 12-31 and 12-32).

The artery follows the dorsal surface of the foot down to the posterior extremity of the first interosseous space, where it crosses vertically to anastomose with the lateral plantar artery. The essential landmark is the tendon of the extensor hallucis longus muscle. Using a bidigital grip, look for the pulse of the dorsalis pedis artery on the dorsum of the foot just lateral to the tendon mentioned above and medial to the tendon of the extensor digitorum longus muscle serving the second toe.

# BIBLIOGRAPHY

# BIBLIOGRAPHY

BEAUTHIER J.-P., LEFEVRE P., *Traité d'anatomie, de la théorie à la pratique palpatoire*. Éd. De Boeck Université, Bruxelles, 1990.

BONNEL F., CHEVREL J.-P., OUTREQUIN G., collection dirigée par J.-P. CHEVREL, *Anatomie clinique, tome 1, Les Membres*. Springer Verlag, Paris, 1991.

BOUCHET A., CUILLERET J., *Anatomie topographique, descriptive et fonctionnelle, Le membre inférieur*. SIMEP éditions, 3e édition, 1996.

DANIELS L., WORTHINGHAM C., *Évaluation de la fonction musculaire Le testing*. Maloine, Paris, 1974.

GUNTZ M., *Nomenclature anatomique illustrée*. Masson, Paris, 1975.

HOPPENFELD S., *Physical examination of the spine and extremities*. Appleton-Century-Crofts edition, New York, 1976.

KAMINA P., *Dictionnaire atlas d'anatomie*. Maloine, Paris, 1983.

KAMINA P., SANTINI J.-J., *Anatomie, introduction à la clinique, nerfs des membres*. Maloine, Paris, 1989.

KENDALL H. O., PETERSON KENDAL F., WADSWORTH G. E., *Les Muscles, bilan et étude fonctionnelle*. Maloine, Paris, 1979.

LACOTE M., CHEVALIER A.-M., MIRANDA A., BLETON J.-P., STEVENIN P., *Évaluation clinique de la fonction musculaire*. Maloine, Paris, 1982.

LAZORTHES G., *Le système nerveux périphérique*. Masson, Paris, 1981.

LOCKHART R. D., *Living anatomy*. Faber and Faber limited, 3e édition, London, 1951.

LUMLEY JOHN S., *Surface anatomy*. Churchill Livingstone, Edinburgh, 1990.

McMINN R. M. H., HUTCHINGS R. T., *Atlas d'anatomie*. Delta & Spes, Denges (Suisse), 1984.

MOLLIER S., *Plastische anatomie*. J. F. Bergmann Verlag, 2e édition, München, Unveränderter Neudruck, 1967.

PIERRON G., LEROY A., PENINOU G., DUFOUR M., GENOT C., *Kinésithérapie 2, membre inférieur*. Flammarion Médecine-Sciences, 1984.

ROUVIÈRE H., DELMAS A., *Anatomie humaine, descriptive, topographique et fonctionnelle*, Tome 3, Masson, Paris, 13e édition, 1991.

ROYCE J., *Surface anatomy*. F. A. Davis Company, USA, 1965.

TESTUT L., JACOB O., *Traité d'anatomie topographique*. Octave DOUIN éditeur, Paris, 1914.

TOBY C., *Methodische palpation*, S. Karger Verlag, Berlin, 1905.

WOLF-HEIDEGGER G., *Atlas des systematischen Anatomie des Menchen*, Vol. III. Basel—Münschen—Paris, S. Karger, 1972.

# INDEX

# INDEX

Abductor digiti minimi muscle, 130, 131, **187**
Abductor hallucis muscle, 130, 131, **188**
Achilles tendon, **121**
  ankle/foot
    anterolateral/anteromedial approach, **181**
    lateral, 131
    medial, 131
  leg
    lateral, 101
    lateral view, 111
    medial, 101
    medial view, 124
    posterior, 100
    posterior view, 116
    posterolateral view, 117
Adductor brevis muscle, **47**
Adductor hallucis muscle, **189**
Adductor longus muscle, **47**
  anterior, 34
  anteromedial view, 37
  medial, 35
  medial view, 46
  sartorius muscle, and, 38
Adductor magnus muscle
  inferior bundle, **48, 89**
  intermediate bundle, **48**
  medial, 35
  posterior (hip), 3
  posterior (thigh), 34
  tendon, 85
  vertical bundle, **48**
Adductor muscles, 39, **47, 48**
Adductor tubercle, **68**
Ankle/foot, 129–194
  abductor digiti minimi muscle, 187
  abductor hallucis muscle, 188
  achilles tendon, 181
  adductor hallucis muscle, 189

annular ligaments of tarsum, 175
anterior calcaneotalar joint, 170
anterior surface of ankle, 152–155
anterior tibialis tendon, 178
arthrology, 164–176
articular interspaces, 164–176
articulation of Chopart, 169
articulation of Lisfranc, 167, 168
calcaneus, 137–139, 150
cuboid bone, 136
cutaneous intermediate dorsal nerve, 192
dorsal aponeurosis of foot, 176
dorsal interossei muscles, 190
dorsal surface of foot, 152–155
dorsalis pedis artery, 194
extensor digitorum brevis muscle, 179, 185
extensor digitorum brevis tendon, 186
extensor digitorum longus tendon, 179
extensor hallucis brevis muscle, 178, 185
extensor hallucis longus tendon, 178
fifth metatarsal bone, 134, 135
first dorsal interosseus muscle, 190
first metatarsal bone, 143–145
flexor digiti minimi brevis muscle, 187
flexor digitorum longus tendon, 182, 183
flexor hallucis brevis muscle, 189
flexor hallucis longus tendon, 183
illustrated study (anterior), 130
illustrated study (dorsum), 130
illustrated study (lateral), 131
illustrated study (medial), 131
interphalangeal joints, 165
intrinsic muscles of foot, 184–190
lateral border, 133–141
lateral malleolus, 141
ligaments of tibiotarsal joint, 173, 174
lumbricales muscles, 190
medial border, 142–151
medial cuneiform bone, 146
medial malleolus, 151
medial tarsal joint, 169

Note: The boldface numbers denote primary in-depth references to the subject area.

Ankle/foot (*Cont.*)
  metatarsophalangeal joints, 166
  musculocutaneous nerve, 192
  musculotendinous structures, 177–183
  myology, 177–190
  navicular bone, 147
  nerves/vessels, 191–194
  opponens digiti minimi muscle, 187
  osteology, 133–163
  peroneus brevis muscle, 180
  peroneus brevis tendon, 180
  peroneus longus muscle, 180
  peroneus tertius tendon, 179
  plantar interossei muscles, 190
  plantar surface, 159–163
  posterior calcaneotalar joint, 170
  posterior surface, 156–158
  posterior tibial artery, 193, 194
  posterior tibial nerve, 193, 194
  posterior tibialis tendon, 182
  posteroinferior tibiofibular ligament, 175
  quadratus plantae muscle, 189
  subtalar joint, 170
  superficial peroneal nerve, 192
  talus, 140, 148, 149
  tarsometatarsal joints, 167, 168
  tibiotarsal joint, 171, 172
  topographic presentation, 132
Annular ligaments of tarsum, **175**
Anterior calcaneotalar joint, **170**
Anterior compartment, 61–65
Anterior talofibular ligament, **173**
Anterior tibialis muscle, 106, **107**
  ankle/foot, 109, 174, 176
    anterior view of ankle, 108
    dorsal view of foot, 108
    tendon, 131, **178**, 193
  knee, 81, **83, 84**
  leg
    anterior, 100
    anterior view, 101
    lateral view, 112, 114
Anterior tibialis tendon, 131, **178**, 193
Anterofemoral region, 37–44
  quadriceps extensor muscle, 40–42
  sartorius muscle, 38, 39
  tensor muscle of the fascia lata, 43, 44
Anteroinferior annular ligament of tarsum, **175**
Anterolateral region, 81–84
Anteromedial region, 85–89
Anterosuperior annular ligament of tarsum, **175**
Anterosuperior iliac spine, 5, **6**
Arthrology. *See also* Joints; Ligament(s)
  ankle/knee, 164–176
  knee, 75–80

Articulation of Chopart, **169**
Articulation of Lisfranc, **167, 168**
ASIS, 2, 34

Biceps femoris muscle, **56**
  knee
    medial, 59
    posterior view, 90
  leg, 101
  long head
    hip (lateral), 2
    hip (posterior), 3
    knee, 58
    lateral, 35
    posterior, 34
    posterior view, 51
    posterolateral view, 55
  short head
    knee, 58
    lateral, 35
    posterior, 34
    posterior view, 51
    posterolateral view, 55
  tendon, 58, 59, 81, **82, 92**, 101, 117
  thigh
    medial, 35
    posterior view (tendon), 45, 51
    posteromedial aspect, 49
Biceps femoris tendon
  knee
    anterior, 58
    anterolateral, 81
    distal aspect, **82**
    lateral, 59
    popliteal fossa, and, **92**
  leg, 101, 117
Bone(s)
  anterior surface of ankle, 152–155
  calcaneus. *See* Calcaneus
  cuboid. *See* Cuboid bone
  dorsal surface of foot, 152–155
  femur. *See* Femur
  fibula. *See* Fibula
  fifth metatarsal. *See* Fifth metatarsal bone
  first metatarsal. *See* First metatarsal bone
  fourth metatarsal, **153**
  iliac. *See* Iliac bone
  lateral malleolus. *See* Lateral malleolus
  lateral sesamoid, **161**
  medial cuneiform, 131, **146**
  medial malleolus. *See* Medial malleolus
  medial sesamoid, **161**
  navicular, **147**
  patella. *See* Patella

plantar surface of foot, 159–163
posterior surface of ankle/foot, 156–158
second metatarsal, **154**
sesamoids, **143, 161**
suprapatellar fossa, **62, 71**
talus. *See* Talus
third metatarsal, **154**
tibia. *See* Tibia

Calcaneal sulcus, 138
Calcaneal (achilles) tendon. *See* Achilles tendon
Calcaneal tuberosity, 100
Calcaneofibular ligament, **173**
Calcaneonavicular ligament, 174
Calcaneotibial bundle, **174**
Calcaneus
    anterior, 130
    anterior surface, **137**
    anterior tubercle of inferior surface, **162**
    cuboid facet, **137**
    floor of sinus tarsi, **138**
    greater process, **137**
    groove of calcaneus, **150**
    lateral, 131
    lateral portion of posterior segment, **139**
    lateral surface, **137**
    leg, 101, 117
    lesser process, **150**
    medial, 131
    peroneal trochlea, **138**
    posterior portion of lateral surface, **139**
    posterior segment of inferior surface, **162**
    posterior segment of superior surface, **158**
    posterior surface, **157**
    sustentaculum, **150**
    tubercle of insertion of calcaneofibular ligament, **139**
Common peroneal nerve, **96, 97**
    lateral, 59
    leg, 101
    popliteal fossa, 93, 94, 95
    posterior, 58
Crest of the tibia, **103**
Cuboid bone
    dorsal surface, **136**
    lateral border, **136**
    plantar surface, **136, 160**
Cuboid facet, **137**
Cutaneous intermediate dorsal nerve, 191, **192**
Cutaneous lateral dorsal nerve, 191, **192**

Deltoid ligament, 131, **174**
Dorsal aponeurosis of foot, **176**
Dorsal interosseus muscles, **190**
Dorsalis pedis artery, 191, 193, **194**

Extensor digitorum brevis muscle, 131, **179, 185**
Extensor digitorum brevis tendons, 130, **186**
Extensor digitorum longus muscle, **110**
    ankle/foot, 109, 175
    anterior, 100
    anterior view of leg, 105
    dorsal view of foot, 108
    lateral, 101
    lateral view of leg, 112, 114
    leg, **83, 84**
    tendons, **110**, 130, 131, **179**, 193
Extensor digitorum longus tendon, **110, 179**
    anterior view, 193
    dorsum, 130
    lateral, 131
    medial, 131
Extensor hallucis brevis muscle, 108, 130, **178, 185**
Extensor hallucis muscle
    ankle/foot, 108, 131
    leg, 100, 101, 105
    tendon, **109**, 130, 176, **178**, 193
Extensor retinaculum, 101, 105
External compartment, 70–74

Femoral artery, 28, **29**
Femoral head, **10**
Femoral nerve, 28, **29**
Femoral triangle, 15–17
Femorotibial articular interspace, **64**
Femur
    hip
        femoral head, **10**
        greater trochanter, **11**
        lesser trochanter, **12**
    knee
        adductor tubercle, **68**
        articular surfaces of medial/lateral condyles, **65**
        lateral border of lateral aspect of lateral
            trochleocondylar articular surface, **71, 72**
        lateral border of suprapatellar fossa, **71**
        lateral epicondyle, **71**
        lateral supracondylar groove, **72**
        lateral trochleocondylar articular surface, **71, 72**
        medial epicondyle, **67**
        medial supracondylar groove, **68**
        medial trochleocondylar articular surface, **68**
        trochleocondylar grooves, **65**
Fibula, 130
    head, 58, **74**, 81, 117
    lateral surface, **104**
    neck, **74**
Fibular collateral ligament, **76**
Fifth metatarsal bone
    anterior surface of ankle, **153**

Fifth metatarsal bone (*Cont.*)
  base, **135**
  dorsal surface of foot, **153**
  head, **134**
  inferior border of shaft, **134**
  lateral surface of shaft, **134**
  styloid process, **135**
  tubercular eminence, **135**
First dorsal interosseus muscle, **190**
First metatarsal bone
  anterior surface of ankle, **154**
  base, **145**
  dorsal surface, **144**
  dorsal surface of foot, **154**
  head (plantar approach), **143**
  inferior border of shaft, **144**
  lateral surface, **144**
  medial, 131
  medial border, **143**
  phalanges (dorsal approach), **143**
  posterior tubercle, **146**
  posterolateral tubercle, **146, 161**
  sesamoid bones (plantar approach), **143**
Flexor digiti minimi brevis muscle, 130, **187**
Flexor digitorum brevis muscle, 130, **189**
Flexor digitorum longus muscle, 124, **125**
  ankle/foot, 131, 183
  leg, 100, 101
  tendon, **182, 183**
Flexor hallucis brevis muscle, 130, **188**
Flexor hallucis longus muscle, 126, **127**
  ankle/foot, 131, 183
  leg, 124
  tendon, 100, 101, **183**
Flexor retinaculum, 100, 101, 131
Floor of the sinus tarsi, **138**
Foot. *See* Ankle/foot
Fourth metatarsal bone, **153**

Gastrocnemius muscle
  knee, 58, 59
  lateral belly, 100
  lateral head, 90, 111, 112, 114, 116, 117, **119**, 120
  leg, 100, 101
  medial belly, 100
  medial head, 58, 90, 111, 116, 117, **118**, 120
Gemellus muscle, **26**
Gluteal aponeurosis, 2, 3
Gluteal fold, 4, 18, 19, 20, 56
Gluteal region
  deep plane, 23–27
  greater sciatic nerve, 30–32
  middle plane, 21, 22
  posterolateral view, 18

  superficial plane, 19, 20
Gluteus maximus muscle, **20**
  hip, 19
    lateral, 2
    posterior, 3
    posterolateral view, 18
  thigh
    posterior, 34
    posteromedial aspect, 49
Gluteus medius muscle, 2, 13, 21, **22**
Gluteus minimus muscle, **24**
Gracilis magnus muscle, 85
Gracilis muscle, 49, **50**
  hip, 3
  knee, 87
    medial, 59
    posterior, 58
    posterior view, 90
  leg, 101
  tendon, 58, **86, 87, 91**, 100, 101
  thigh
    adductor muscles, and, 48
    anterior, 34
    anteromedial, 37
    medial, 35
    medial view, 46
    posterior, 34
    posterior view, 45, 51
    sartorius muscle, and, 38
Greater saphenous vein, 191, 193
Greater sciatic nerve, 30–32
Greater sciatic notch, **9**
Greater trochanter, 5, **11**, **25**, 30
Groove of the calcaneus, **150**

Hamstring muscles
  lateral, 55, 56
  medial, 52–54
Hip, 1–32
  femoral triangle, 15–17
  femur, 10–12
  gluteal region, 18–27
  greater sciatic nerve, 30–32
  iliac bone, 6–9
  iliofemoral region, 5–12
  illustrated study (lateral), 2
  illustrated study (posterior), 3
  lateral inguinofemoral region, 13, 14
  medial inguinofemoral region, 15–17
  myology, 13–27
  nerves/vessels, 28–32
  osteology, 5–12
  Scarpa's triangle, 15–17
  topographic presentation, 4

Iliac bone
  anterosuperior iliac spine, **6**
  greater sciatic notch, **9**
  iliac crest, **6**
  inferior border of iliac bone, **9**
  ischial spine, **8**
  ischial tuberosity, **9**
  lesser sciatic notch, **8**
  posteroinferior iliac spine, **7**
  posterosuperior iliac spine, **7**
  pubic tubercle, **7**
  small coxal notch, **7**
  tubercle of iliac crest, **6**
Iliac crest, 2, 3, 5, **6**
Iliofemoral region
  femur, 10–12
  iliac bone, 6–9
Iliopsoas muscle, 34, 37, 38
Iliotibial band, 43, **44**, 81, 90
Iliotibial tract
  hip
    lateral, 2
    posterior, 3
  knee
    lateral, 59
    posterior, 58
  thigh
    anterior, 34
    lateral, 35
    posterior, 34
Illustrated studies
  ankle/foot (anterior), 130
  ankle/foot (dorsum), 130
  ankle/foot (lateral), 131
  ankle/foot (medial), 131
  hip (lateral), 2
  hip (posterior), 3
  knee (anterior), 58
  knee (lateral), 59
  knee (medial), 59
  knee (posterior), 58
  leg (anterior), 100
  leg (lateral), 101
  leg (medial), 101
  leg (posterior), 100
  thigh (anterior), 34
  thigh (lateral), 35
  thigh (medial), 35
  thigh (posterior), 34
Inferior extensor retinaculum, 100, 101, 130, 131
Inferior gemellus muscle, **26**
Inferior peroneal retinaculum, 101
Infrapatellar adipose tissue, **80**
Interior inferior annular ligament of tarsum, 193
Interosseus, **143**

Interphalangeal joints, **165**
Ischial spine, **8**
Ischial tuberosity, **9**, 30

Joints
  anterior calcaneotalar, **170**
  articulation of Chopart, **169**
  articulation of Lisfranc, **167**
  dorsal aponeurosis of foot, **176**
  interphalangeal, **165**
  medial tarsal, **169**
  metatarsophalangeal, **166**
  posterior calcaneotalar, **170**
  subtalar, **170**
  tarsometatarsal, **167, 168**
  tibiotarsal, **171, 172**

Knee, 57–98
  anterior compartment, 61–65
  anterolateral region, 81–84
  anteromedial region, 85–89
  external compartment, 70–74
  illustrated study (anterior), 58
  illustrated study (lateral), 59
  illustrated study (medial), 59
  illustrated study (posterior), 58
  ligaments, 75–80
  medial compartment, 66–69
  myology, 81–92
  nerves/vessels, 93–98
  osteology, 61–74
  posterior region, 90–92
  topographic presentation, 60

Lateral annular ligament of tarsum, **175**
Lateral Chopart, **169**
Lateral condyle of tibia, **73**
Lateral epicondyle of femur, **71**
Lateral hamstring muscle, **55, 56**
Lateral inguinofemoral region, 13, 14
Lateral malleolar facet, **171**
Lateral malleolus
  ankle/foot, 130, 131
  anterior border, **141**
  apex, **141**
  leg, 100, 101, 117
  posterior border, **141**
  posterior surface, **158**
Lateral malleolus (tibia), 100
Lateral patellar retinaculum, **76, 77**
Lateral process, **163**
Lateral sesamoid bone, **161**
Lateral supracondylar groove, **72**

Lateral tibial plateau, **73**
Lateral trochleocondylar articular surface, **71, 72**
Leg, 99–127
   achilles tendon, 121
   anterior muscular group, 105–110
   anterior tibialis muscle, 106, 107
   extensor digitorum longus muscle, 110
   extensor hallucis longus muscle, 109
   flexor digitorum longus muscle, 124, 125
   flexor hallucis longus muscle, 126, 127
   illustrated study (anterior), 100
   illustrated study (lateral), 101
   illustrated study (medial), 101
   illustrated study (posterior), 100
   lateral muscular group, 111–115
   myology, 105–127
   osteology, 103, 104
   peroneus brevis muscle, 114, 115
   peroneus longus muscle, 112, 113
   peroneus tertius muscle, 110
   plantaris muscle, 121
   posterior muscular group, 116–127
   posterior tibialis muscle, 122, 123
   topographic presentation, 102
   triceps surae muscle, 117–120
Lesser saphenous vein, 58
Lesser sciatic notch, **8**
Lesser trochanter, **12**
Ligament(s)
   annular ligaments of tarsum, **175**
   anterior talofibular, **173**
   calcaneofibular, **173**
   deltoid, **174**
   fibular collateral, **76**
   infrapatellar adipose tissue, **80**
   interior inferior annular ligament of tarsum, 193
   lateral patellar rectinaculum, **76, 77**
   medial patellar rectinaculum, **77, 79, 80**
   patellar, **80**
   posterior talofibular, **173**
   posteroinferior tibiofibular, **175**
   tibial collateral, **78, 79**
   tibiotarsal joint, of, **173, 174**
Lumbrical(es) muscles, 130, **190**

Maissiat's band, **82**
Medial Chopart, **169**
Medial compartment, 66–69
Medial cuneiform bone, 131, **146**
Medial epicondyle of femur, **67**
Medial hamstring muscles, **52–54**
Medial inguinofemoral region, 15–17
Medial malleolar facet, **172**
Medial malleolus
   ankle/foot, 130

   anterior border, **151**
   inferior extremity, **151**
   leg, 100
   posterior border, **151**
   posterior surface, **151**
Medial patellar retinaculum, **77, 79, 80**
Medial process, **163**
Medial retromalleolar groove, **125, 127**
Medial sesamoid bone, **161**
Medial supracondylar groove, **68**
Medial tarsal joint, **169**
Medial tibial plateau, **69**
Medial trochleocondylar articular surface, **68**
Metatarsal heads, **153, 160**
Metatarsal interspace, **143**
Metatarsophalangeal joints, **166**
Muscle(s)
   abductor digiti minimi, 130, 131, **187**
   abductor hallucis, 130, 131, **188**
   adductor brevis, **47**
   adductor hallucis, **189**
   adductor longus. *See* Adductor longus muscle
   adductor magnus. *See* Adductor magnus
      muscle
   adductor, 39, **47, 48**
   anterior tibialis, 106, **107**
   biceps femoris, **56**
   dorsal interosseus, **190**
   extensor digitorum brevis, 131, **179, 185**
   extensor digitorum longus. *See* Extensor digitorum
      muscle
   extensor hallucis brevis, 108, 130, **178, 185**
   extensor hallucis. *See* Extensor hallucis muscle
   first dorsal interosseus, **190**
   flexor digiti minimi brevis, 130, **187**
   flexor digitorum brevis, 130, **189**
   flexor digitorum longus. *See* Flexor digitorum longus
      muscle
   flexor hallucis brevis, 130, **188**
   flexor hallucis longus. *See* Flexor hallucis longus
      muscle
   gastrocnemius. *See* Gastrocnemius muscle
   gemellus, **26**
   gluteus maximus, **20**
   gluteus medius, 2, 13, 21, **22**
   gluteus minimus, **24**
   gracilis magnus, 85
   gracilis. *See* Gracilis muscle
   hamstrings, 52–56
   iliopsoas, 34, 37, 38
   inferior gemellus, **26**
   lateral hamstring, **55, 56**
   lumbrical(es)s, 130, **190**
   Maissiat's band, **82**
   medial hamstrings, **52–54**

obturator lateralis, **27**
obturator medialis, **26**
opponens digiti minimi, **187**
pectineus, 34, 37, 38, 39, 46, **47**
peroneus brevis. *See* Peroneus brevis muscle
peroneus longus. *See* Peroneus longus muscle
peroneus tertius. *See* Peroneus tertius muscle
pes anserinus, **86–88**
piriformis, **25, 26**
plantar interossei, **190**
plantaris. *See* Plantaris muscle
popliteus, **92**
posterior tibialis. *See* Posterior tibialis muscle
quadratus femoris, **27**
quadratus plantae, **189**
quadriceps extensor, **40–42**, 43, 81
rectus femoris. *See* Rectus femoris muscle
sartorius. *See* Sartorius muscle
semimembranosus. *See* Semimembranosus muscle
semitendinosus. *See* Semitendinosus muscle
soleus. *See* Soleus muscle
superior gemellus, **26**
tensor fascia lata. *See* Tensor muscle of the fascia
    lata
tibialis anterior, 58, 101
triceps surae, **117–120**
vastus lateralis. *See* Vastus lateralis muscle
vastus medialis. *See* Vastus medialis muscle
Musculocutaneous nerve, **192**
Myology. *See also* Muscle(s)
    ankle/foot, 177–190
    hip, 13–27
    knee, 81–92
    leg, 105–127
    thigh, 37–56

Navicular bone, **147**
Nerves and vessels
    ankle/foot, 191–194
    cutaneous intermediate dorsal nerve, 192
    dorsalis pedis artery, 194
    femoral artery, **29**
    femoral nerve, **29**
    hip, 28–32
    knee, 93–98
    musculocutaneous nerve, 192
    peroneal nerve. *See* Common peroneal nerve
    popliteal artery, 93, **98**
    popliteal fossa, **93–98**
    posterior tibial artery, 193, 194
    posterior tibial nerve, 193, 194
    superficial peroneal nerve, 192
    sural nerve, 95, **97**
    tibial nerve, 93, 94, **95**

Oblique crest, **74**
Obturator lateralis muscle, **27**
Obturator medialis muscle, **26**
Opponens digiti minimi muscle, **187**
Osteology. *See also* Bone(s)
    ankle/foot, 133–163
    hip, 5–12
    knee, 61–74
    leg, 103, 104

Patella
    anterior surface, **62**
    apex, **63**
    base, **62**
    hip, 34, 35
    knee, 58, 59, 81
    lateral approach to posterior surface, **63**
    lateral borders, **63**
    leg, 101
    medial approach to posterior surface, **64**
Patellar ligament, 40, 58, 59, **80**, 81, 100, 101
Patellar retinaculum, 59
Pectineus muscle, 34, 37, 38, 39, 46, **47**
Peroneal malleolar facet, **171**
Peroneal nerve. *See* Common peroneal nerve
Peroneal trochlea, **138, 158**
Peroneus brevis muscle, 114, **115**
    ankle/foot, 108, 131, **180**
    leg, 100, 101, 111, 112, 117, 120
    tendon, 100, **180**
Peroneus longus muscle, 112, **113**
    anterior, 100
    knee, 58, 59
    lateral, 101
    lateral view, 111, 114
    leg, **83, 84**, 120
    tendon, 100, 117, 120, 131, **180**
Peroneus tertius muscle, **110**
    ankle/foot, 108
    leg, 105
    tendon, 130, 131, 175, **179**
Pes anserinus muscles, **86–88**
Piriformis muscle, **25, 26**
Plantar interossei muscles, **190**
Plantaris muscle, **121**
    knee, 59
    lateral, 101
    posterior, 100
    posterior view, 116
    posterolateral view, 117
    tendon, 100
Popliteal artery, 58, 93, **98**
Popliteal fossa, **93–98**
Popliteal vein, 58
Popliteus muscle, **92**

Posterior calcaneotalar joint, **170**
Posterior region, 90–92
Posterior talofibular ligament, **173**
Posterior talotibial bundle, **174**
Posterior tibial artery, 191, 193, **194**
Posterior tibial nerve, 193, **194**
Posterior tibialis muscle, 122, **123**
   ankle/foot, 183
   medial view, 124
   tendon, 100, 126, 174, **182**
Posterior tibialis vein and artery, 100
Posterior tuberosities, 162, **163**
Posterofemoral region, 45–56
   adductor muscles, 47, 48
   gracilis muscle, 49, 50
   lateral hamstring muscle, 55, 56
   medial hamstring muscles, 52–54
   medial muscular group, 46–50
   posterior muscular group, 51–56
Posteroinferior iliac spine, **7**
Posteroinferior tibiofibular ligament, **175**
Posterosuperior iliac spine, **7**
Pubic tubercle, **7**

Quadratus femoris muscle, **27**
Quadratus plantae muscle, **189**
Quadriceps extensor muscle, **40–42**, 43, 81
Quadriceps femoris, 59
Quadriceps femoris tendon, 58

Retinaculum
   extensor, 101, 105
   flexor, 100, 101, 131
   inferior extensor, 100, 101, 130, 131
   inferior peroneal, 101
   lateral patellar, **76, 77**
   medial patellar, **77, 79, 80**
   patellar, 59
   superior peroneal, 100, 101, 131
Rectus femoris muscle, **14, 42**
   hip
      anterolateral view, 21
      anteromedial, 13
      lateral, 2
   knee, 81
   thigh
      anterior, 34
      anterior view, 40
      anterolateral view, 43
      anteromedial view, 37
      lateral, 35
      medial, 35
      medial view, 46
      sartorius muscle, and, 38, 39

Sartorius muscle, 38, **39**
   hip, **14**, 16
      anteromedial view, 13
      lateral, 2
      medial view, 15
   knee
      distal aspect, 86, **88**
      medial, 59
      posterior, 58
   leg, 101
   tendon, 58, 100
   thigh
      anterior, 34
      anterior view, 40
      anterolateral view, 43
      anteromedial view, 37
      lateral, 35
      medial, 35
      medial view, 46
      posterior, 34
      relationship to other thigh muscles, 38
Scarpa's triangle, 15
Sciatic nerve, 30–32
Second metatarsal bone, **154**
Semimembranosus muscle, **54, 91**
   knee
      lateral, 59
      medial, 59
      medial view, 85
      posterior, 58
      posterior view, 90
   leg, 100
   tendon, **88**, 101
   thigh
      lateral, 35
      medial, 35
      posterior, 34
      posterior view, 45, 51
      posterolateral view, 55
      posteromedial aspect, 49
      posteromedial view, 52
Semitendinosus muscle, **53**
   hip, 3
   knee
      medial, 59
      posterior, 58
      posterior view, 90
   tendon, 45, 85, 86, **87, 91**, 100, 101
   thigh
      medial, 35
      posterior, 34
      posterior view, 51
      posterolateral view, 52, 55
      posteromedial aspect, 49
Sesamoid bones, **143, 161**

Sinus tarsi, **138**
Small coxal notch, **7**
Soleus muscle, **120**
  anterior, 100
  knee, 58, 59
  lateral, 101
  lateral view, 111, 112, 114
  medial, 101
  posterior, 100
  posterior view, 116
  posterolateral view, 117
Subtalar joint, **170**
Sulcus tali, **138**
Superficial peroneal nerve, 191, **192**
Superior gemellus muscle, **26**
Superior peroneal retinaculum, 100, 101, 131
Suprapatellar fossa, **62, 71**
Sural nerve, 95, **97**
Sustentaculum tali, **150, 157**

Talar trochlea, **171, 172**
Talus
  lateral process, **140**
  lateral surface of neck, **140**
  lateral tubercle, **149**
  ligamentous field/middle field of head, **148**
  medial portion of neck, **148**
  medial tubercle, **149**
  neck, **155**
Tarsometatarsal joints, **167, 168**
Tendon(s)
  achilles. *See* Achilles tendon
  adductor magnus, 85
  anterior tibialis, 131, **178**, 193
  biceps femoris, 58, 59, 81, **82**, **92**, 101, 117
  extensor digitorum brevis, 130, **186**
  extensor digitorum longus, **110**, 130, 131, **179**, 193
  extensor hallucis, **109**, 130, 176, **178**, 193
  flexor digitorum longus, **182, 183**
  flexor hallucis longus, 100, 101, **183**
  gracilis, 58, **86, 87, 91**, 100, 101
  iliotibial tract, of, **82**
  peroneus brevis, 100, **180**
  peroneus longus, 100, 117, 120, 131, **180**
  peroneus tertius, 130, 131, 175, **179**
  plantaris, 100
  posterior tibialis, 100, 126, 174, **182**
  quadriceps femoris, 58
  sartorius, 58, 100
  semimembranosus, **88**, 101
  semitendinosus, 45, 85, 86, **87, 91**, 100, 101
  tibialis anterior, 130, 131
  tibialis posterior, 101
Tensor muscle of the fascia lata
  hip, **14**

  anterolateral view, 14
  anteromedial view, 13
  lateral, 2
  posterior, 3
  thigh, 43, **44**
    anterior, 34
    anterior view, 40
    anterolateral view, 43
    anteromedial view, 37
    lateral, 34
    medial view, 46
    sartorius muscle, and, 39
Thigh, 33–56
  adductor muscles, 47, 48
  anterior muscular group, 37–44
  anterofemoral region, 37–44
  gracilis muscle, 49, 50
  illustrated study (anterior), 34
  illustrated study (lateral), 35
  illustrated study (medial), 35
  illustrated study (posterior), 34
  lateral hamstring muscle, 55, 56
  medial hamstring muscles, 52–54
  medial muscular group, 46–50
  myology, 37–56
  posterior muscular group, 51–56
  posterofemoral region, 45–56
  quadriceps extensor muscle, 40–42
  sartorius muscle, 38, 39
  tensor muscle of the fascia lata, 43, 44
  topographic presentation, 36
Third metatarsal bone, **154**
Tibia
  ankle/foot
    anterior border of lower extremity, **155**
    dorsum, 130
    medial, 131
  head, 59, 100, 101
  knee
    anterior, 58
    anterior tuberosity, **64**
    inferior border of medial condyle, **69**
    medial, 59
    proximal aspect of medial border, **69**
    tubercle of Gerdy, **73**
  leg
    anterior, 100
    anterior border, **103**, 105
    lateral surface, 104
    medial, 101
    medial border, 103
    medial surface, 104
    posterior surface, 104
  oblique crest, **74**
Tibial collateral ligament, **78, 79**

Tibial malleolar facet, **172**
Tibial nerve, 58, 93, 94, **95**, 100, 191
Tibial plateau, **64, 69, 73**
Tibial tuberosity, 58, 59, 81, 100, 101
Tibialis anterior muscle, 58, 101
Tibialis anterior tendon, 130, 131
Tibialis posterior tendon, 101
Tibionavicular bundle, **174**
Tibiotarsal joint, **171–174**
Topographic presentations
  ankle/foot (anterolateral view), 132
  ankle/foot (anteromedial view), 132
  hip (anterolateral view), 4
  hip (posterolateral view), 4
  knee (anterior view), 60
  knee (posterior view), 60
  leg (anterior view), 102
  leg (posterior view), 102
  thigh (anterior view), 36
  thigh (posterior view), 36
Triceps surae muscle, **117–120**
Trochleocondylar grooves, **65**
Tubercle of Gerdy, **73**
Tubercle of iliac crest, 5, **6**
Tubercle of insertion of calcaneofibular ligament, 139
Tuberosity of the fifth metatarsal bone, **153**

Vastus lateralis muscle, **41, 82**
  hip, 2
  knee
    anterior, 58

    anterolateral view, 81
    lateral, 59
  thigh
    anterior, 34
    anterior view, 40
    anterolateral view, 43
    anteromedial view, 37
    lateral, 35
    medial view, 46
    sartorius muscle, and, 39
Vastus medialis muscle, **41, 89**
  knee
    anterior, 58
    anterolateral view, 81
    medial, 59
    medial view, 85
    muscular body, **89**
  thigh
    anterior, 34
    anterior view, 40
    anterolateral view, 43
    anteromedial view, 37
    medial, 35
    medial view, 46
    posterior view, 51
    posteromedial aspect, 49
    sartorius muscle, and, 38, 39
Vessels. *See* Nerves and vessels

"Y" ligament of medial tarsal joint, **169**

# NOTES